7 READ THE SMALL PRINT AND THE BIG WORDS

Ingredient labels tell you what is inside.
Pick items with words that sound like food, not science.
Always ask yourself: Is this a **SUPER ME GRRR8** choice?

8 LIMIT FOODS THAT AREN'T HELPING

Every Bite Matters. A little salt, sugar or fatty food is ok. Make a goal to only eat them **once a week.**

9 MAKE MORE ME TIME

Recharge your batteries - turn off the tech.
Make more time to sing, dance, learn, read, cook, discover and 8-9 hours of sleep.

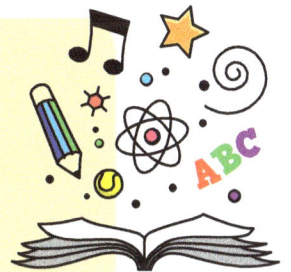

11 LISTEN TO YOUR BODY

Foods can make some people feel sick.
If your body hurts, tell an adult.
You might need a food allergy test.

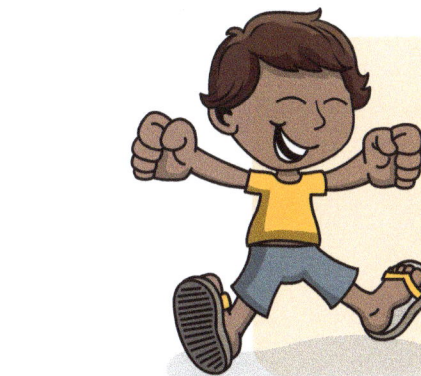

10 DREAM

Dream with a goal and never give up.

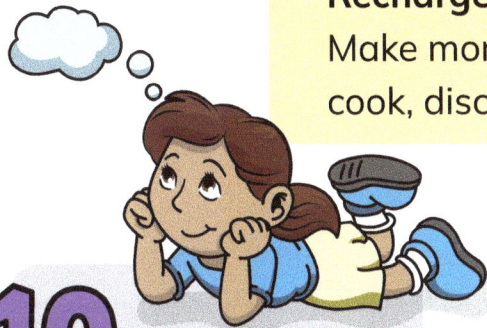

12 OWN HAPPY

Focus on good things to help power your smile. Try to make every day a great day. If life causes you to feel yucky, you are not alone. **Talk to an adult that makes you feel safe and strong.**

Scientists say smiling can help people feel happy.
This makes the people around them feel happier, too!
So, put a bounce in your step. Let your eyes twinkle and your mouth smile.

MAKE YOUR WORLD A HAPPY PLACE.

I0106090

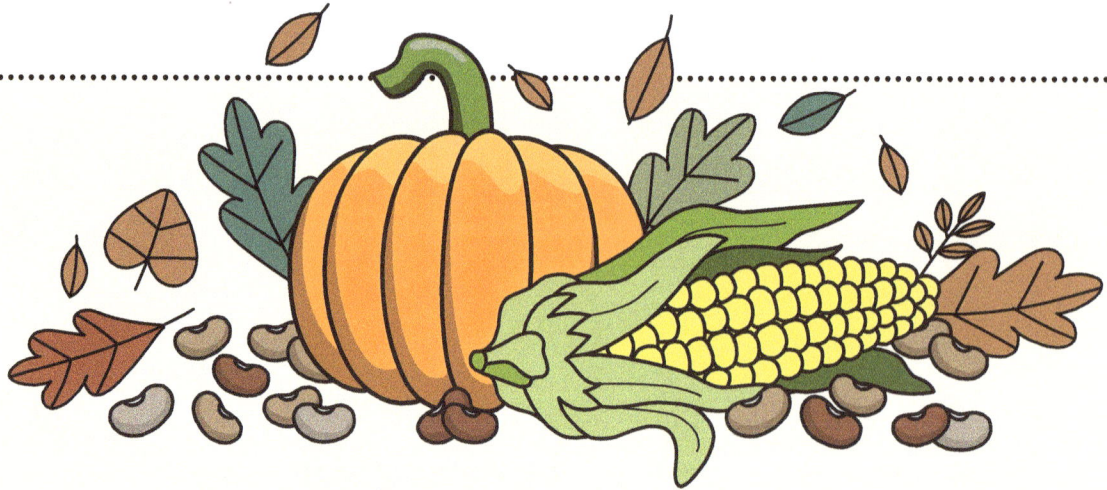

"Empowering our youth to understand how their choices determine their future health and wellbeing improves the quality of life for each person, family and community."

National Center for Chronic Disease Prevention and Health, 2022

SUPER ME ®

Ben B. You are the #1 Super Me Champion!
The nearly two year Covid lockdown hit you hard. Once free, you decided to become your own force for Happy Heart change. As a 3rd grader, you created Healthy Happy Heart Tricks all on your own. You upped your daily fitness activity and cut out all that wasn't helping you grow strong and healthy. You are amazing. You are my inspiration.

A huge thank you goes to Sanja Kostić for designing this beautiful and fun educational book. You fill every page with love.

Thank you to my reviewers and experts: Cyd, Debbie, Dorothy, Jen, Nina, Lori, Christina, Ricardo, and Dominika. Your input makes this project GRRR8. Thank you: Cary, Sarah and Jim for making sure I get an A+ for grammar and spelling.

Jurgen, you always lead by example - keep running and eating oats.

No part of this book may be copied or transmitted without written permission from Walnut Canyon Press.

Library of Congress Control Number: 2023933795
©2023 Walnut Canyon Press
Printed in the U.S.A

PERFECT PEOPLE PORTIONS

Use your handy dandy hand for the perfect tool to measure food.

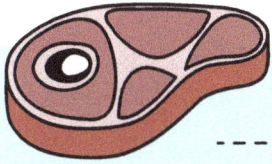

BUTTER
One fingertip-sized amount of butter for one piece of bread.

MEAT
Your palm and no thicker than your pinky finger = one serving.

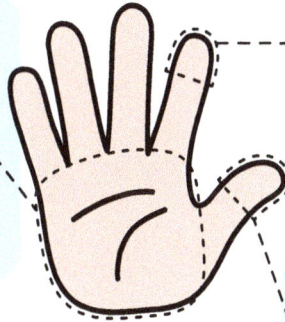

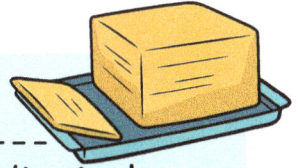

NO SUGAR PEANUT BUTTER
Two thumbs = one serving.

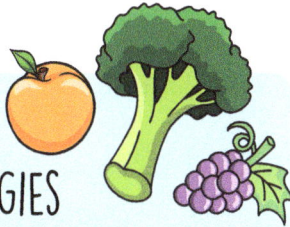

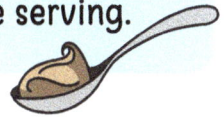

FRUITS AND VEGGIES
One serving = one fist
Remember: You need five servings in a day.

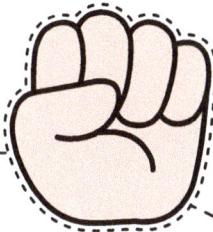

DAIRY
One serving = one fist
Remember: You need three to four in a day.

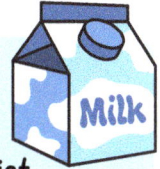

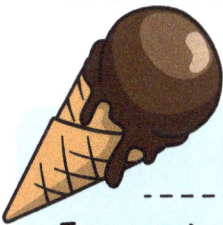

ICE CREAM
Two servings = your fist!
Half a fist = one serving.

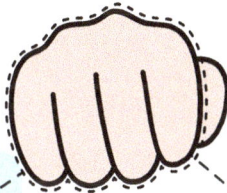

PASTA
Dry pasta:
one clenched fist.
Cooked pasta:
one open handful.

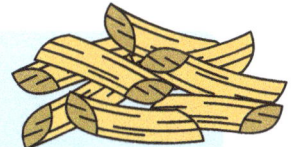

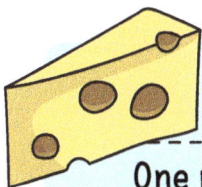

CHEESE
One portion = about two fingers.

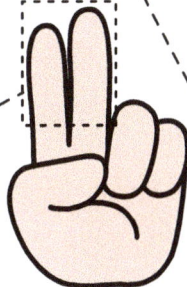

SAD HEART CARBS
Your cupped hand = bread, muffin, cake or cookies.

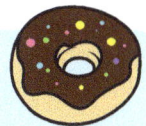

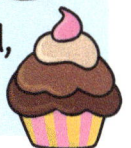

THIS BOOK BELONGS TO:

_____

Dear Super You,

Super Me is an adventure FULL of GRRR8 clues which can help you and your family feel GRRR8 and stay healthy.

Enjoy activities that make it fun to be smart. Discover how everything connects.

Learn how doing well in school and growing a strong body has lots to do with your smallest everyday choices.

Learn **Happy Healthy Heart** tricks that save your family money.

Travel the world with GRRR8 QR code links hiding on the pages. (Remember: always ask the adult in charge, before you click!)

Ask someone older to read the 'Letter to the Home Team" on page 117. Ask them to be part of your Super Me Dream Team.

Just two Super Me pages a day or one chapter a week and some cooking will help keep you fit and GRRR8.

America needs SUPER GRRR8 kids to grow up and take care of our country. Let these fun tricks help you on your journey to become your

SMARTEST, STRONGEST, MOST SUPER AMAZINGLY GRRR8 YOU!

Let's BE GRRR8 as we swing into this adventure together!

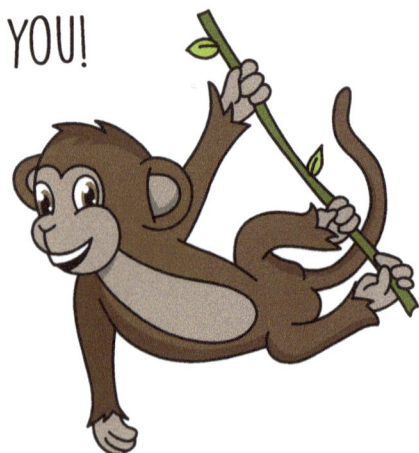

SUPER WEEKLY FUN — CHALLENGE YOURSELF TO GET IT DONE!

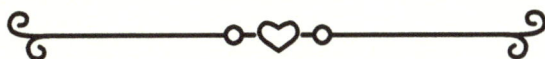

I WILL SUCCEED!

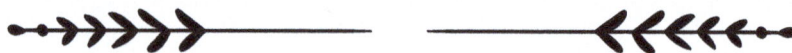

•••→→>>> ——— ——— <<<←←••

"Every great dream begins with a dreamer. Always remember, you have within you the strength, the patience and the passion to reach the stars to change the world." — Harriet Tubman

Draw what you will look like when you grow up:

When I grow up I will be: ....

Why? Because: ....

....

....

....

....

CHECK IT OUT!

HEALTHY CHOICES
FOR ME TO SUCCEED

Below are some choices you will make in the next nine or ten years.
Pick the ones you believe are most important for your success.
Write them below. Cross out the choices you think won't help.

Things I can do as I grow to help keep me on my GRRR8 path are:

....

....

....

....

....

....

....

....

....

....

| Help in school. | Love the library. | Dream. | Be the best student I can be. |

| Eat healthy food. | Learn all I can. | Play lots of games. | Eat lots of candy. |

| Drink lots of soda. | Drink lots of water. | Eat 5 fruits and veggies every day. |

| Do all my homework. | Exercise every day. | Stay up late. | Read lots of books. |

| Learn everything I can on interesting subjects. | Get 8 hours of sleep each night. |

| Come to school each day prepared to give my best. | Forget to do my homework. |

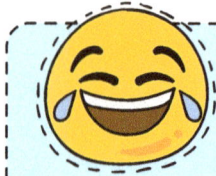

SUPER ME
A Healthy Outside Starts Inside.

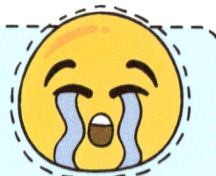

I have the power to control what I think and how I feel inside.
All that goes on outside and around me is temporary.

Connect the happy face to all the things you can control.
Shrug off those things you can't and cross them out.

How I Feel

How others treat me

Take care of my health

My time

How I react to unkindness

Laugh!

Focus on my goals

What others say

My friendships

What others do

Know right from wrong

Love myself

Sleep enough

My ideas

Drink water

Ask for help

Choices I make

My time

What others think

Dance!

How others behave

Moving and grooving

Sing!

How I treat others

The past

Talk to an adult,
if I don't feel safe

Read

How I treat myself

My future

Not letting others
hurt my feelings

Know that bad things
are never forever

Focus on a good attitude,
even when life feels pretty bad.

How I learn and grow

What I eat

Help others

Think about things I
wish were different

Work hard in school

Find ways to be happy

How I spend my time

What I think

People who are mean to me

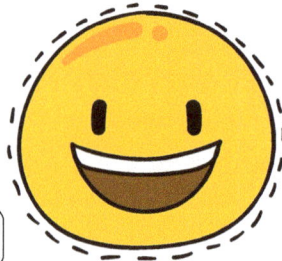

HOW WELL DID I HELP CARE FOR MY BODY TODAY?

My healthy checklist for every day of the week.

	Mon	Tue	Wed	Thu	Fri	Sat	Sun
I laughed, danced, jumped and smiled today.							
I ate less salt, sugar and fat filled food.							
I drank enough water.							
I slept at least 8 hours.							
I exercised at least 30 minutes.							
I washed my hands after using the bathroom, coming home from school, before cooking and eating.							
I made the best Happy Healthy Heart food choices I could today.							
I ate 5 vegetables and fruit servings!							
I brushed my teeth at least 2 times.							
I learned something new today.							
I listened to my body.							
I was proud of myself.							
I was thankful for something.							
I focused on good thoughts.							
I was kind.							

A GREAT START FOR A BEAUTIFUL NEW DAY

"Morning, my angels! It is a beautiful new day.
Come on, sleepy heads - the early bird catches the worm,"
sings Mom, as she wakes my brother and me.

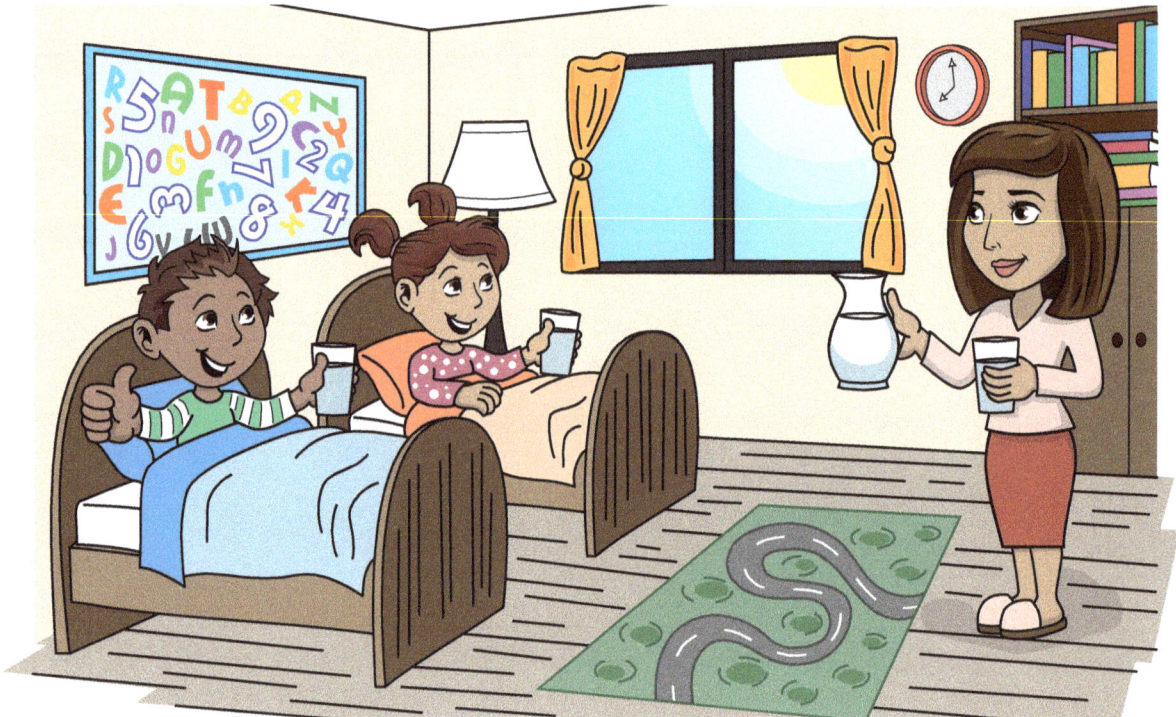

"Here's your water. Just like plants, we need lots of water to grow, especially after sleeping. Here's a new riddle," Mom says. ***"What runs but never walks? WATER!"***

She laughs as she gives us our water, already enjoying herself.

Mom loves water. Any time we feel a bit icky, sad, tired, grouchy, headachy, her first question is always:

"Did you drink enough water today?"

"Mom, loves water so much, maybe she should marry water!"

"Look, a dead bug."

"That bug, ... must not have drunk enough water!"

"You are right, I LOVE WATER!!!" Mom laughs. "Clean drinkable water is a very precious thing. Over 800 million people - that is more than everyone in all of the USA, Canada and Mexico combined - do not live near drinkable water. Imagine not being able to go to school because you have to walk all day to carry home water."

"Now hurry up! It is time for breakfast. First one down gets to make the main dish!" Mom chuckles as she walks away.

We drink our water and get ready to start our newest GRR8 day.
Ready? Set? Go! We race into the kitchen.

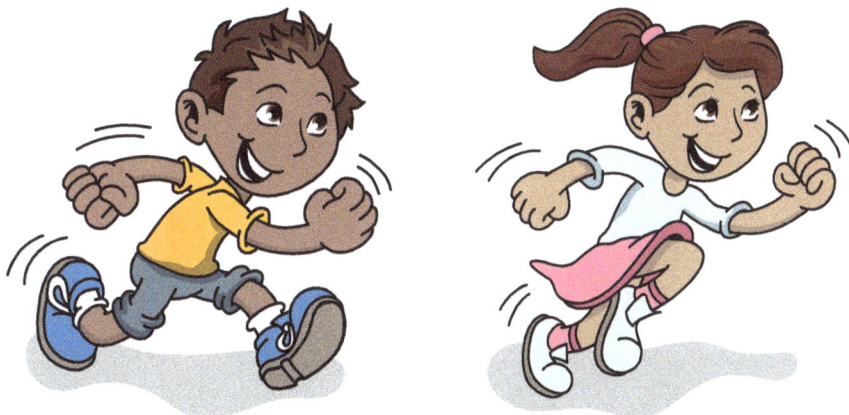

CHECK IT OUT!

FUN IN THE SUN

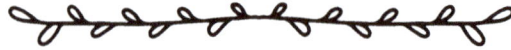

Fill in the rhyming words below to finish the poem. Color in the picture. Draw a picture of yourself having fun!

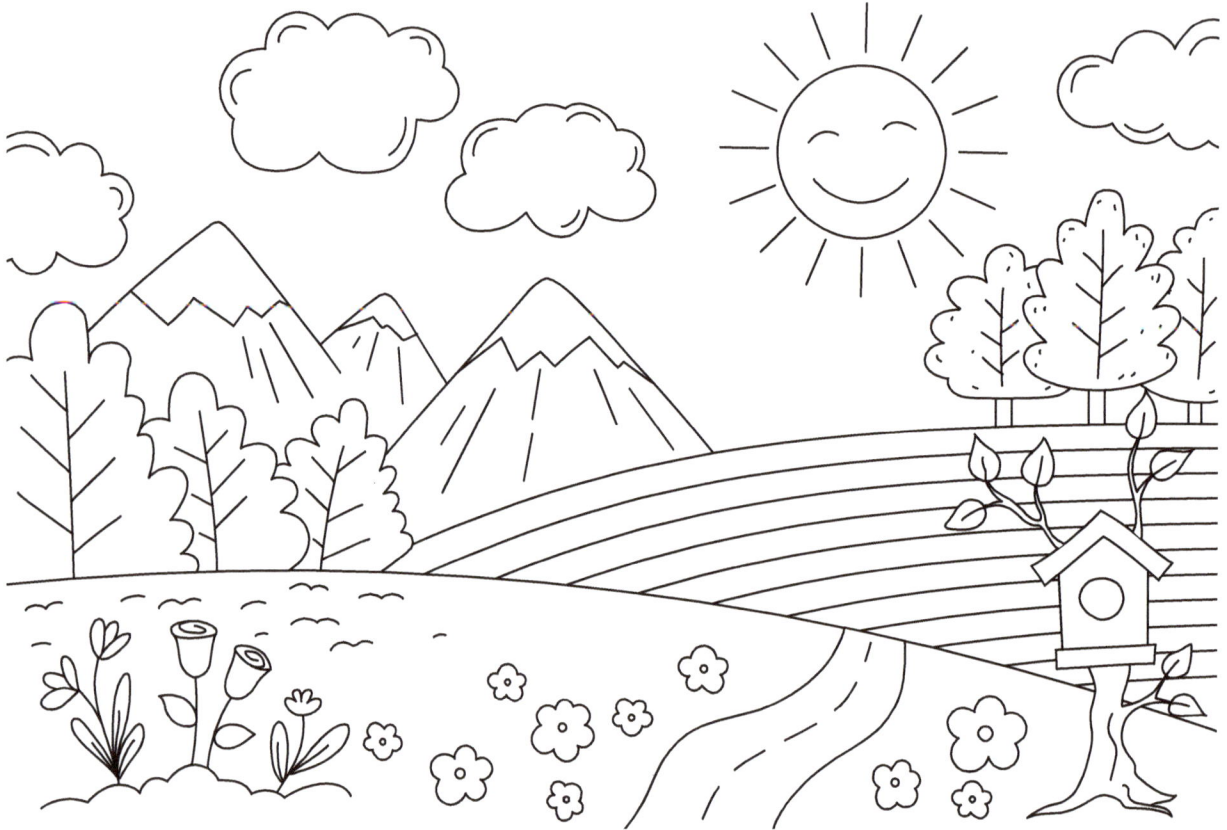

In the morning, I wake and look out at the ....

What will I do to make the day ....

I can hop, skip, jump, or ....

Or maybe, I will count backward, four, three, two,...

Before I know it, the day is ....

I head home for dinner, and eat a hot ....

WORD BANK
One, Moon, Run, Soon, Fly, Sun, Over, Fun, Done, Sandwich, Bun, Zero, Sky

Draw a picture of your favorite fruit or vegetable.
Check the internet to learn why it is GRRR8 for you.
Write your discoveries below.

....

....

....

....

....

....

EASIEST, SMARTEST AND BEST HEALTH TRICK?
DRINK WATER

The number of 8-ounce servings of water we need each day depends on lots of things like body type, amount of exercise and weather.

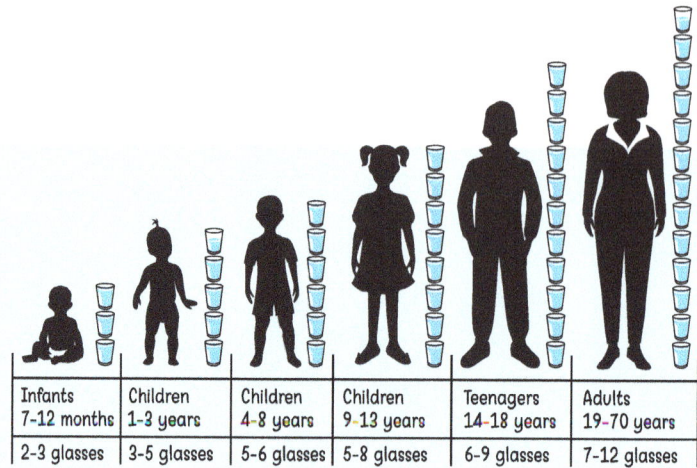

Infants 7-12 months	Children 1-3 years	Children 4-8 years	Children 9-13 years	Teenagers 14-18 years	Adults 19-70 years
2-3 glasses	3-5 glasses	5-6 glasses	5-8 glasses	6-9 glasses	7-12 glasses

One 8-ounce cup = the size of a single milk box serving.

Use the chart above to see how many cups of water you, friends and family members should drink each day.

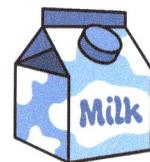

TIPS to drink more water:

- Drink sugar-free juice in very small glasses.

- Add water to drinks and juices. Each time, try to add a little more water.

- Add a slice of cucumber or fruit to a glass of water for your very own fancy drink. It tastes great.

- Keep reusable water bottles filled to grab as you rush out the door. This tiny tip is HUGE! It helps save money and the planet.

Name	Age	Cups of water each day

WATER LOG ▷ LOVE WATER — DRINK WATER!

Record everything you drink. Each week total the amount in each group. Are you getting the right amount of water per day? How many cups of juice and soda do you drink?

Challenge yourself to drink more water and milk, less juice and soda. Remember: Juice and soda can have the same amount of sugar.
Try drinking more water and milk. **Eat Fruit - Drink Water!**

Week:	1	2	3	4	1	2	3	4	1	2	3	4	1	2	3	4
What?	Water				Milk				Juice				Soda			
Monday																
Tuesday																
Wednesday																
Thursday																
Friday																
Saturday																
Sunday																
Total cups:																

Week One: .... ✔   Week Two: .... ✔

Week Three: .... ✔   Week Four: .... ✔

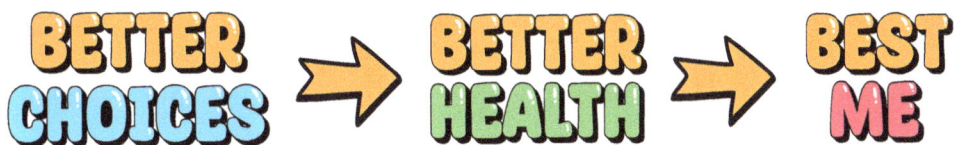

BETTER CHOICES → BETTER HEALTH → BEST ME

CHECK IT OUT!

6

I AM HOW MUCH WATER?

Help Water Our Body Parts!

Color up to the percent (%) line showing how much water is in each body part. Fill in the amounts (round up or down) in the blue boxes.

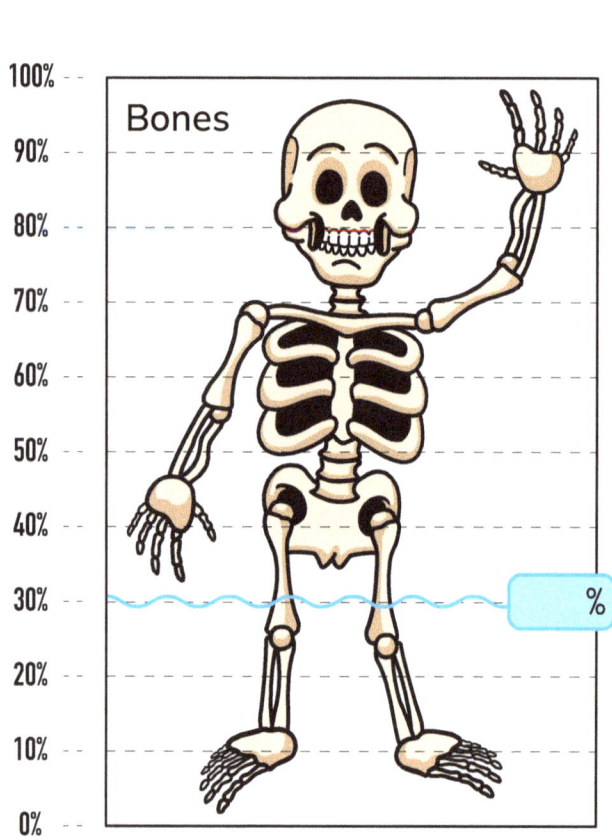

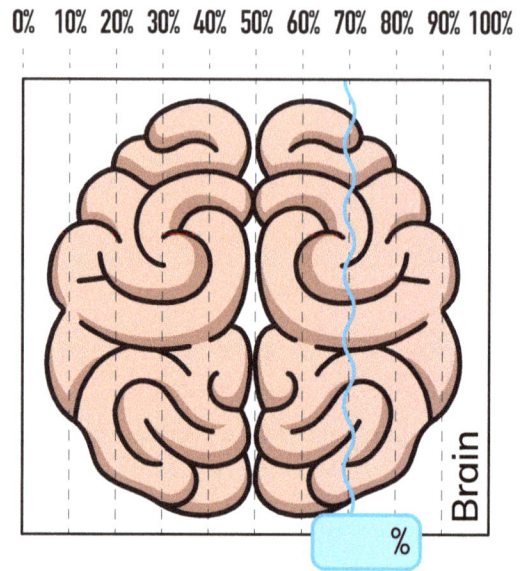

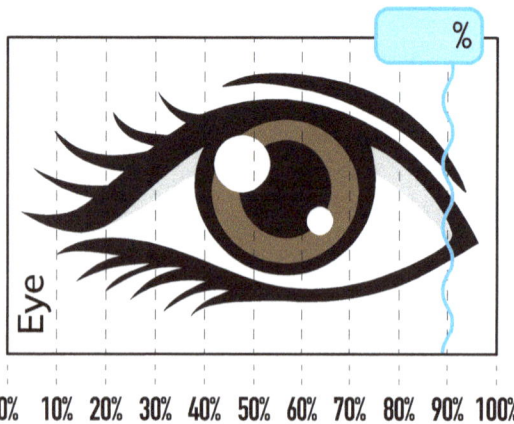

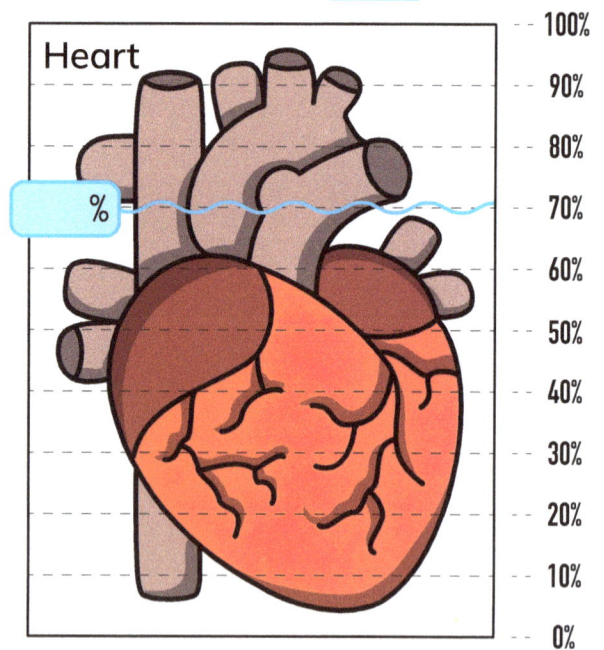

Bones

Brain

Heart

Eye

CHECK IT OUT!

Answers: Eye: 98% Bones: 31% Brain & Heart 73%

BREAKFAST LIKE A BEAR

"Eat breakfast like a bear, lunch like a llama, and dinner like a duck."

"That's funny. Why eat like a bear for breakfast and a duck for dinner? Isn't it better to eat like a bear all the time?" I wondered.

"Actually, that would be very unhealthy. Not all meals should be the same. Our bodies need different amounts of food at different times," Big Brother (BB) explains.

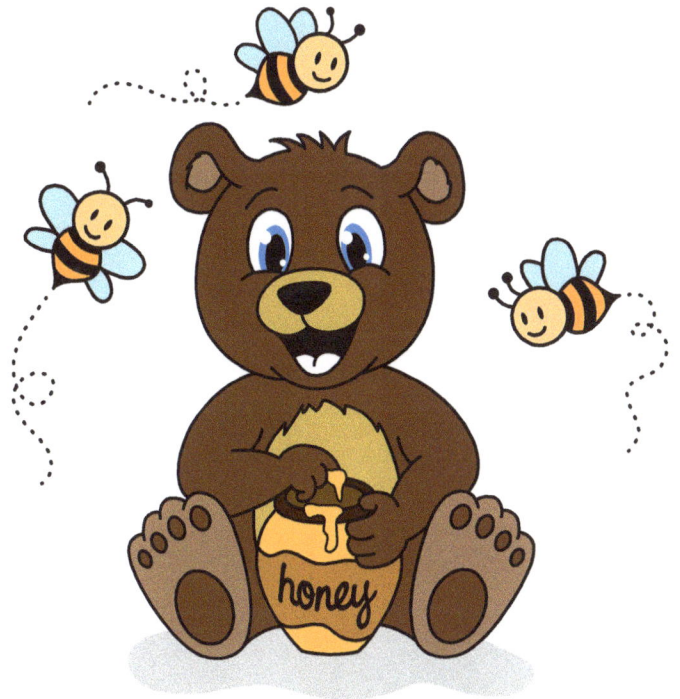

"Hey Sis, Why didn't the teddy bear finish his breakfast?"

"He was stuffed!"

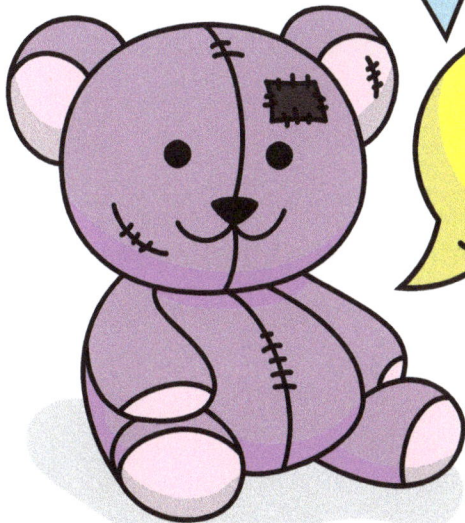

"Breakfast is the most important meal of the day.

After a long sleep, we need to start up our engines. The better we feed our bodies in the morning, the better we do in school.

'Breakfast Like a Bear' means our biggest meal should be breakfast."

*"**Happy Healthy Heart** food keeps us strong, healthy and smart. We need to be smart about fueling our brains and our bodies. You can't drive a car without gas, right?"* Says BB.

Mr. Science doesn't stop. It is a good thing I like to learn, because he is always explaining.

"Each morning our metabolism* needs good fuel to start our engines."

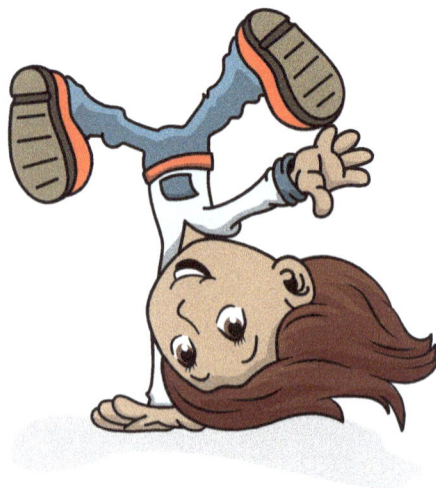

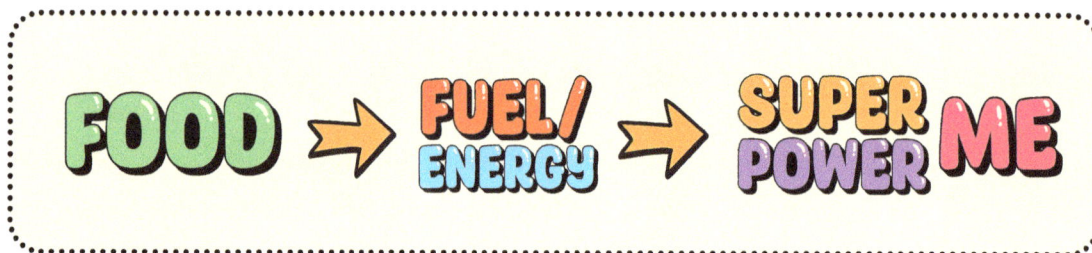

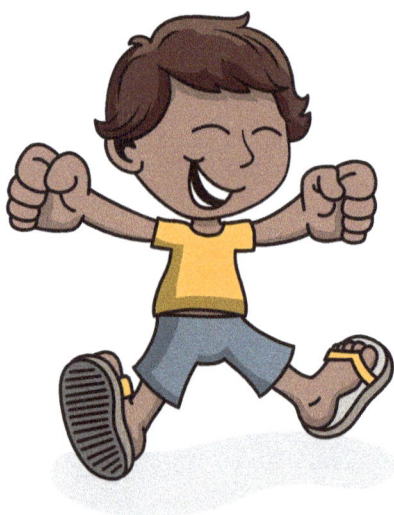

FOOD ⟹ **FUEL/ ENERGY** ⟹ **SUPER POWER ME**

A **Happy Healthy Heart** *breakfast fuels our body so all of our switches turn on, supercharging us for a GRRR8 morning.*

Eating the wrong things or skipping breakfast doesn't give the body enough SUPER ME power. Sugary or fatty foods turn into more fat.

This causes us to feel lazy, move slowly, or stay sleepy. It is harder to understand, think, remember and learn. This means really smart people can feel like a snail or sound confused.

*(meh-**TAB**-uh-liz-um) When the cells in our body change food into energy.

CHECK IT OUT!

During the day, we need good quality food and water to keep us running at our best.

By lunch, a lot of heavy thinking is behind us. We still need good fuel to power the rest of the day.

"Lunch Like a Llama" means we still need to eat really healthy food, only not as much.

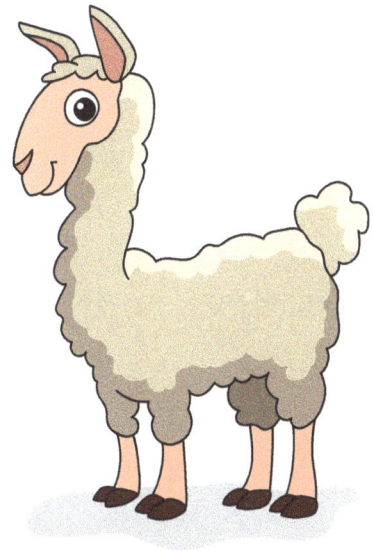

"The evening is the time for homework, gentle stretching, dreaming and sleeping.

'Dinner Like a Duck' means eating a light, easily digestible meal.

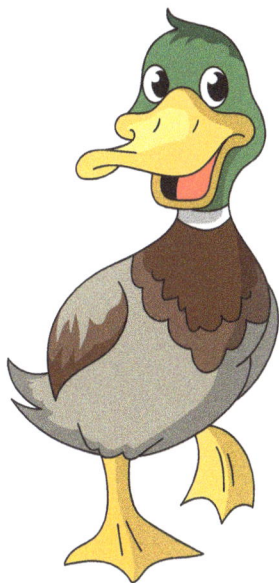

Foods that have a lot of fat or grease like burgers and fries are very hard for the body to digest. Light meals of fruits, vegetables, eggs, oats, quinoa, or chicken are easier to digest because they have lots of fiber and are low in fat. Not only does this let us sleep better, our organs and our metabolism get to rest, too."
BB explains.

What did the mayo say to the mustard?

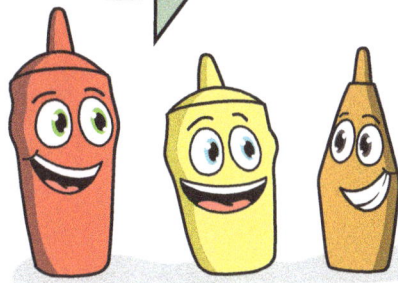

"It has been such a long time. Let's get together, so we can ketchup."

CHECK IT OUT!

BEARS LOVE HONEY AND SO SHOULD YOU

Bees make honey. Honey has been a food and medicine for centuries. Honey can last a really long time. Archaeologists* found 3,000-year-old honey. It was still delicious!

Many people use honey for healing. A teaspoon of honey in warm water can help soothe coughs, sore throats and swallowing.

Honey is a better sweetener choice than regular sugar but should still be used moderately.

Honey is only safe for kids older than two years old.

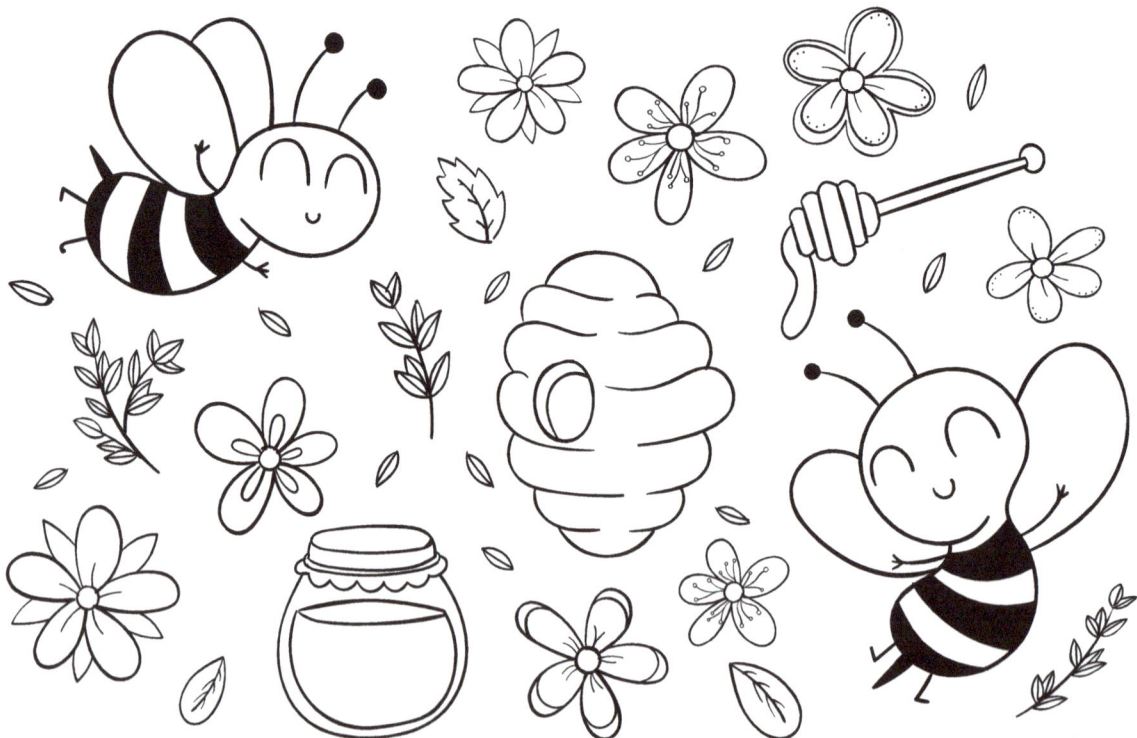

*(ark-ee-**ALL**-oh-gist) someone who studies discoveries found in ancient excavation sites.

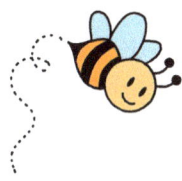

HONEYCOMB ART

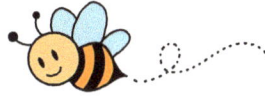

Bees live in hives or colonies.

They build hexagonal wax cells for their larvae* and the queen, and to store their food (honey and pollen). This is called a honeycomb.

Create a honeycomb art pattern below. Repeat as many colors and shapes as you like. You can combine little cells into one larger shape.

Have fun!

❋ START WITH A HEALTHY BREAKFAST ❋

Each morning, we all help make a solid **Happy Healthy Heart** breakfast.

This is usually oatmeal, quinoa* or eggs. Together, we cut fruit and veggies.

We pour cold glasses of plant-based or regular milk.

The whole time we ask questions, help each other practice our lessons for school or just say silly things like...

"What did the raisin say to the oatmeal on Valentine's Day?

"Say, she ate oatmeal... She would be healthy!" Get it? Satiate?**

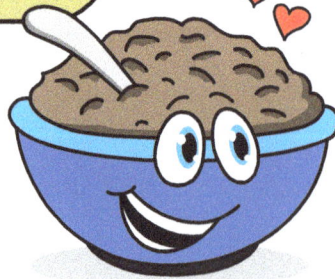

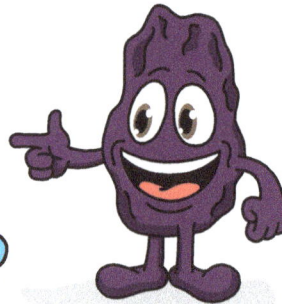

"Oh, you are SOOO mushy!"

Oatmeal is a Super GRRR8 Heart Helper.
It keeps our hearts and blood healthy.
It keeps our intestines clean, too.
Eating oatmeal can help people lose weight, fight asthma and diabetes.
Soaked in water, oats help calm itchy skin and rashes.

DID YOU KNOW?

*Quinoa (**KEY**-nwah) looks like rice but it is really a Super-GRRR8 protein.
(SAY**-she-ate) means fills you up and keeps you full for a long time.

CHECK IT OUT!

My brother LOVES oatmeal. He is always talking about why oatmeal is one of the best foods on the entire planet. Of course, BB has great reasons to love oatmeal. Oatmeal is full of protein, minerals, antioxidants, fiber and vitamins and it costs about 60 cents for an adult-sized serving.

"You can eat it hot or cold, cooked or raw. Oatmeal satiates* and is easy to make," he happily explains to anyone listening.

TRICK

Super Duper - in a Hurry - Fresh Oatmeal
Time to make: 2 minutes

At night, put a handful or two of oats in a jar. Cover with water or milk.
Add a spoon of no-sugar nut butter or some honey. Store them in the fridge.

To eat: heat in the microwave for one minute or eat cold.
If you like, add a smashed banana, some fruit, nuts or raisins.

Prepackaged Instant vs. Raw Oatmeal

THINK ABOUT IT!

Are both as healthy? Can you read the ingredients in both?
Are there fats, sugars or salt hiding in the package?
Which is the smartest choice for a Happy Healthy Heart? Why?
Which lets you save a whole lot of money, your health and the planet (less cost, less 'extra ingredients' & less packaging)?

I LOVE EGGS

The egg is a super food because it is one of the healthiest foods on the planet. Eggs help keep all our systems happy, healthy and working at top speed.

This extremely healthy source of body building GRRR8ness costs about 25 cents, depending on where you live.

HEALTHY ORGANS = SUPERPOWERS!

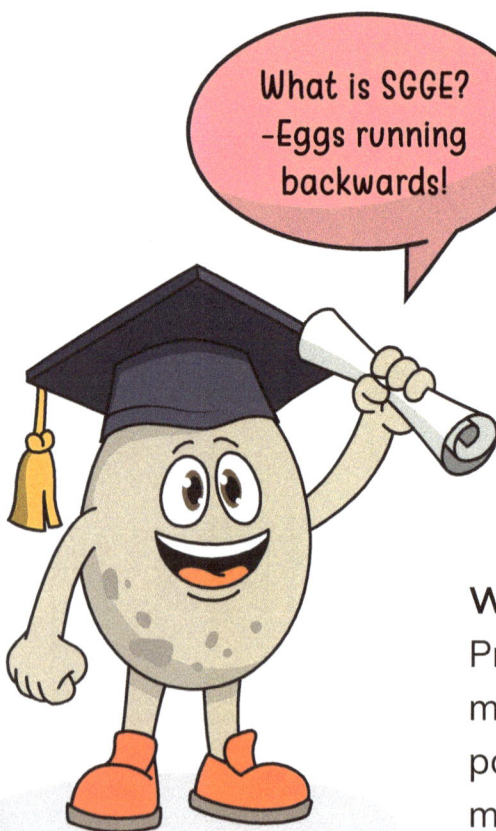

What is SGGE?
-Eggs running backwards!

What is the maximum number of eggs you can eat on an empty stomach? One. After that, your stomach isn't empty!

Why did the rooster and the hen send their eggs to school? They wanted them egg-u-cated!

What's in an Egg?

Protein, calcium, vitamins, fiber, good fats, minerals, nutrients, folate, antioxidants, potassium, choline, selenium, all amino acids, manganese, biotin, vitamins A, B1, B2, B3, B5, B6, B12, D, E and zinc.

OLD MCDONALD HAD A FARM...

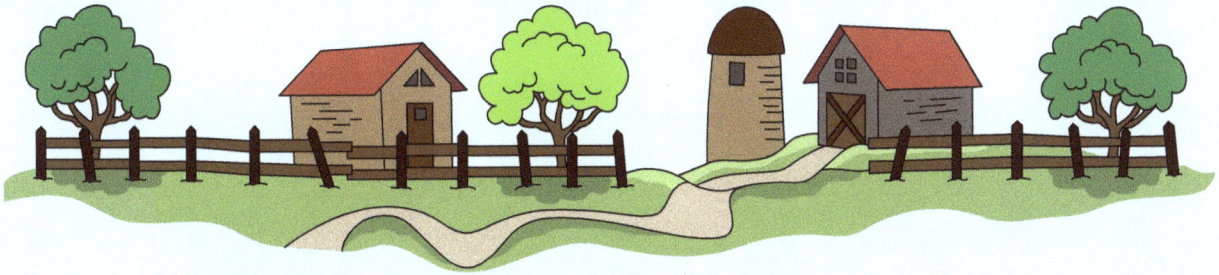

Mr. MacD has one rooster and five hens. Every day, each hen lays one egg. (Roosters don't lay eggs.) Using different colors, draw the number of eggs each chicken lays in one week. Circle groups of 12 eggs.

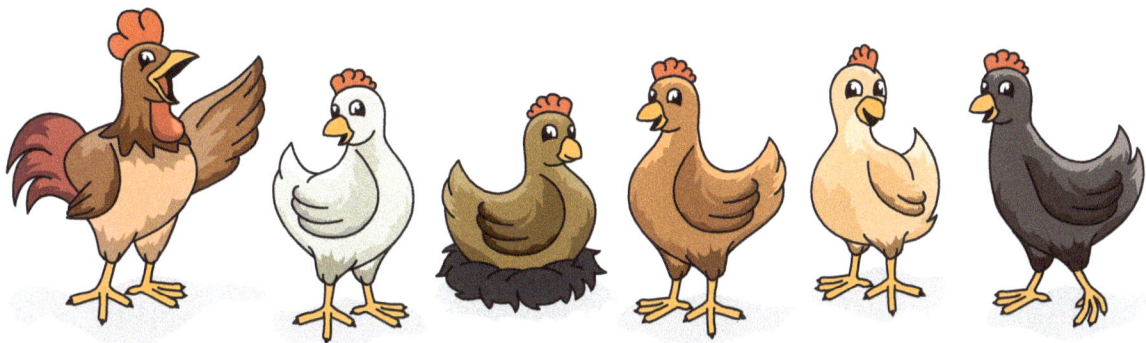

How many eggs will Old MacDonald have in one week?

[ ] eggs **X** [ ] days **=** [ ] eggs

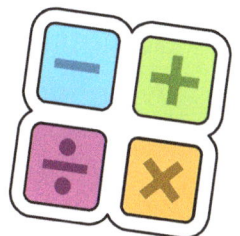

Each egg sells for 10 cents. How much does he earn in one week?

[ ] eggs **X** [ ] cents **=** $ [ ]

How many dozens will he take to market? (1 dozen= 12)

[ ] dozen **+** [ ] remaining

CHECK IT OUT!

BUSY AS BUMBLEBEES IN THE KITCHEN

My brother and I have been helping in the kitchen since we were tiny. We started mixing and measuring. We learned about cups (c.), pints (pt.), quarts (qt.), gallons (gal.), ounces (oz.), teaspoons (tsp.), tablespoons (tbs.) and pounds (lb.). We learned that most other countries use grams (g.), liters (l.) and kilos (kg.).

Sometimes when we cook, we use recipes. Sometimes we experiment. We always have fun.

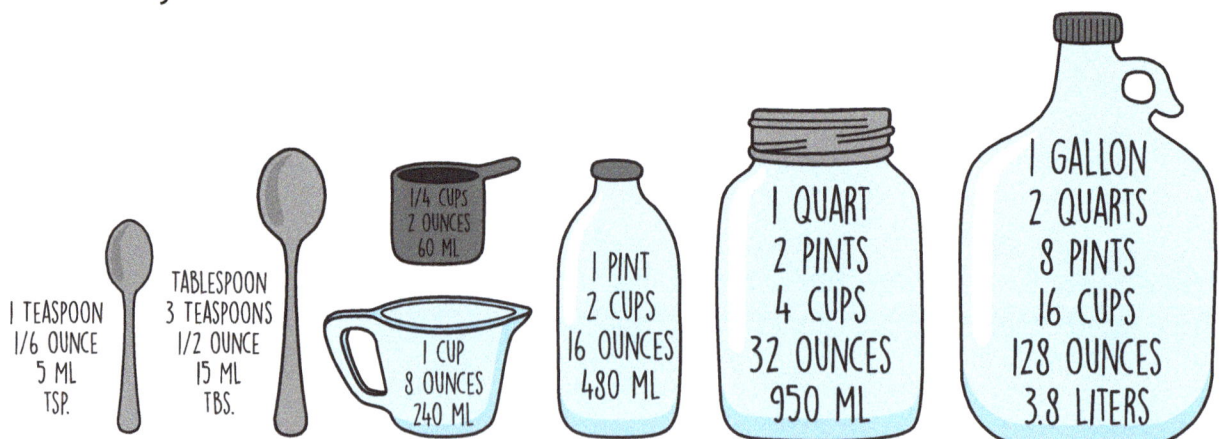

1 TEASPOON
1/6 OUNCE
5 ML
TSP.

TABLESPOON
3 TEASPOONS
1/2 OUNCE
15 ML
TBS.

1/4 CUPS
2 OUNCES
60 ML

1 CUP
8 OUNCES
240 ML

1 PINT
2 CUPS
16 OUNCES
480 ML

1 QUART
2 PINTS
4 CUPS
32 OUNCES
950 ML

1 GALLON
2 QUARTS
8 PINTS
16 CUPS
128 OUNCES
3.8 LITERS

This morning, I am cooking eggs. My brother puts out healthy tortillas, beans, chopped vegetables, salsa and milk for strong bones. Working together, it only takes a few minutes to get everything ready.

Looking at all the beautiful edible modern art on our table makes me smile. I know the pretty crunchy colors full of protein, vitamins, amino acids and minerals help keep us healthier and smarter.

We sit together, laughing, chatting, eating yummy, crunchy, GRRR8 food. I think this is the best way to start the day.

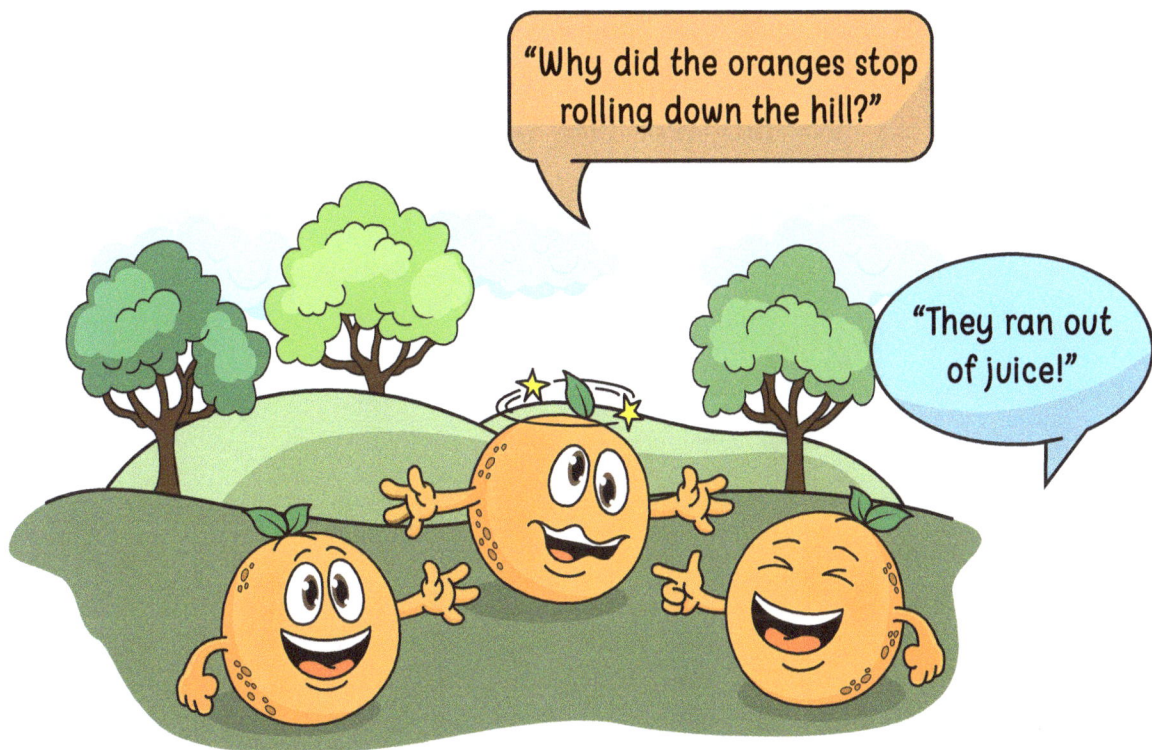

How many oranges does it take to make one glass of juice?
About 4 oranges = One 8 oz glass of juice = about 6 teaspoons of sugar.

Pure fruit juice has a lot of sugar and has all the fiber removed. This much of any kind of sugar is hard on your body.

Eat fruit. Drink water.

THINK ABOUT IT!

CHECK IT OUT!

MAKE A JUICY, CRUNCHY COLOR WHEEL

The bright colors of fruits and vegetables are antioxidants. Antioxidants* reduce damage to our cells. This keep us healthy and fights things like cancer, heart disease, stroke and other diseases.

Red, blue and yellow are called **primary** colors.
Mixing primary colors together makes **secondary** colors.
Purple, green and orange are secondary colors.

Color in the fruits and vegetables.

Use a primary color over the primary triangle = △

Use a secondary color to trace over the secondary color = △

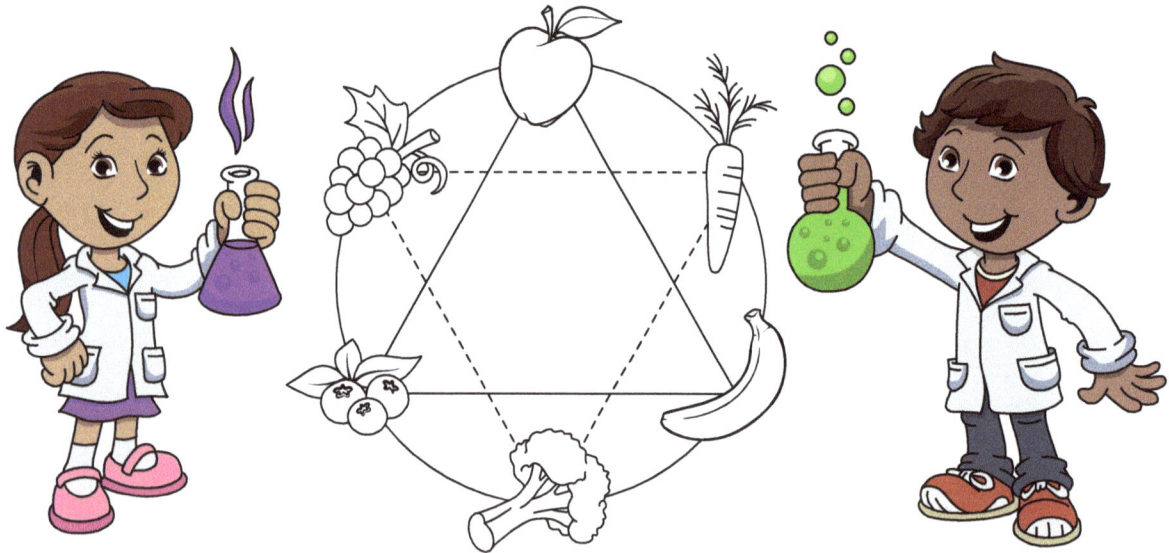

What other fruits and vegetables have:

Primary color antioxidants?

....

....

....

....

Secondary color antioxidants?

....

....

....

....

* (an-tee-**OX**-sa-dent)

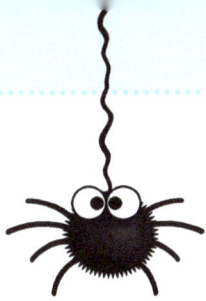

SPIDER'S WEB

Think of a new word or phrase you have learned. Draw spaces for each letter in the box below. Leave empty spaces if using more than one word.

Have someone pick letters to guess the word or phrase. You can give a hint explaining why this is important to be GRRR8. Each time a letter is guessed, cross it out in the alphabet row below.

Fill in all the spaces with each correct guess. Every time they miss, draw a body part. **Remember** - a spider has 8 legs, a body, 2 eyes, and a mouth.

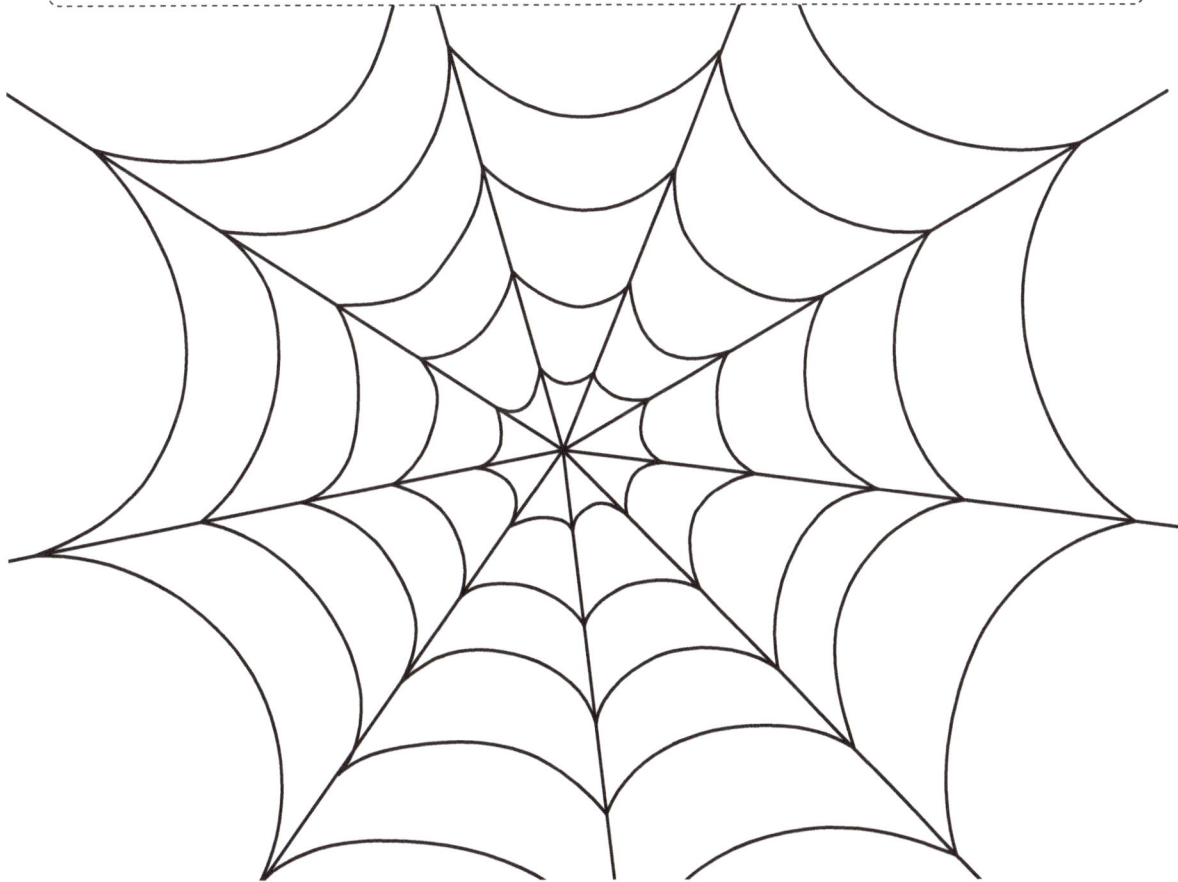

A B C D E F G H I J K L M N O P Q R S T U V W X Y Z

LUNCH LIKE A LLAMA

After finishing breakfast, BB and I make our lunches.

Made@Home Happy Healthy Heart lunches keep us smart and strong. We make them ourselves, so they are always yummy. We make things like smashed beans on whole grain bread, a hard boiled egg and tortilla, unsweetened yogurt with oats and applesauce or quinoa salad.

Celery stuffed with nut butter or cream cheese and raisins are "Ants on a Log" (p.89). We pack something crunchy, like apples, celery, peas, jicama or carrots. These yummy, juicy, sweet, great big vitamin filled treats with are handy-dandy-good-for-your-teeth toothbrushes on the go!

Of course, we always bring a refillable water bottle.

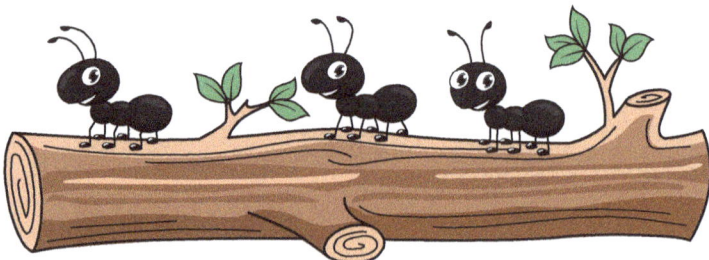

Refilling 4 water bottles a day is free and keeps 1460 plastic bottles from being made, transported and out of the trash, each year.

You save money and the planet! **DID YOU KNOW?**

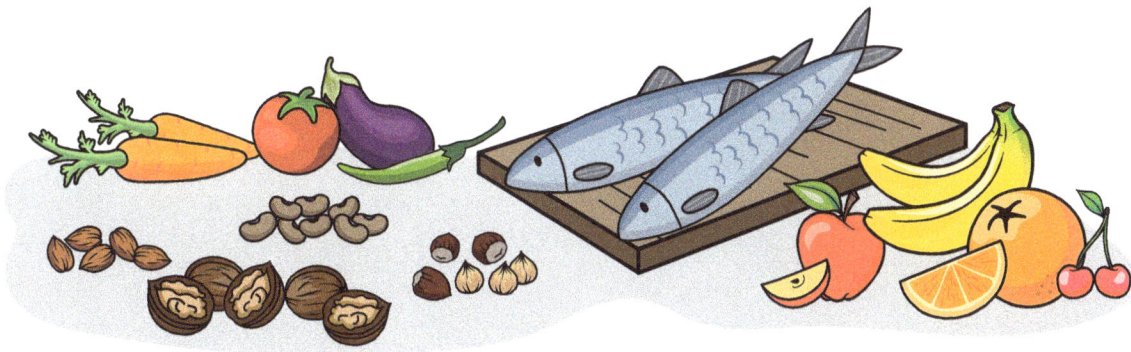

Top athletes are very careful to keep fit. They drink lots of water, eat **Happy Healthy Heart** food and exercise every day.

Since school is our job, we need to do the same thing. We make SUPER GRRR8 lunches so we can be SUPER GRRR8! This helps us be smart, keep our blood pumping and our heart happy. Beans, grains, seeds, fish, lean meats, nuts, brightly colored vegetables and fruit are stuffed with goodness.

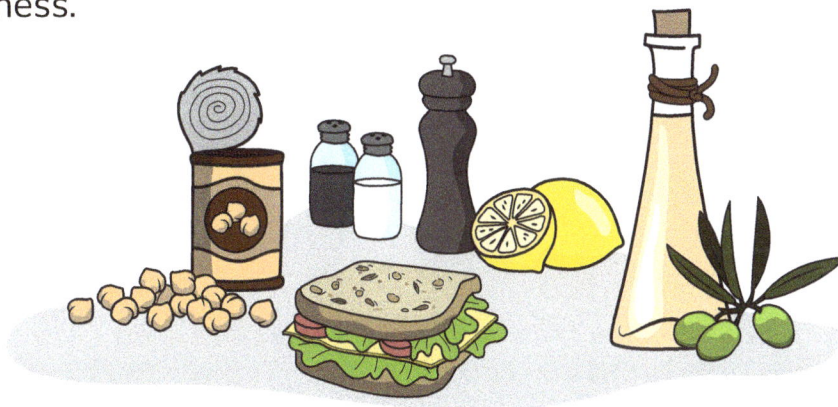

Super Power Packed Meal? **BEANS!**

Beans are Healthy Happy Heart smart. They are packed with protein, vitamins, fiber and they keep our blood stable.

Scientists say two cups of beans per week lower the chances of diseases like cancer, heart issues and diabetes.

Beans and tortillas or bread is as perfect as it gets.

So much GRRR8 for so little $!

DID YOU KNOW?

CHECK IT OUT!

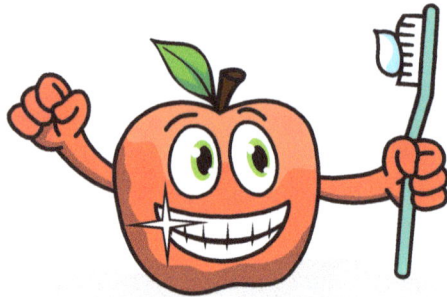

"An apple a day keeps the doctor away... and it helps keep the dentist away, too!"

My doctor told me that for many people, the choices we make can help or even cause some types of diabetes*.

Since Grandma has diabetes, I could get diabetes, as well. This makes it extra important for my family to pay attention to our life choices. We help our bodies by exercising every day and knowing every bite matters.

We eat mostly **Happy Healthy Heart** plant-based foods. They satiate and give us more fiber to keep our insides clean. Whole grain breads, tortillas, rice have lots of fiber. Factory food usually has little good things like vitamins and fiber but lots of salt, sugar and fat, so we rarely eat these.

Everyone knows it is important to respect our teachers and other students. We must also respect ourselves and our bodies. These wellness changes make it easier for our bodies to stay healthy and balanced.

POWER FOODS = POWER HEALTH = $ SAVED

Fiber is only found in plants.
Fiber makes us feel full. It keeps our digestive system clean by moving food efficiently through our body. This is why eating foods from plants is so important.

DID YOU KNOW?

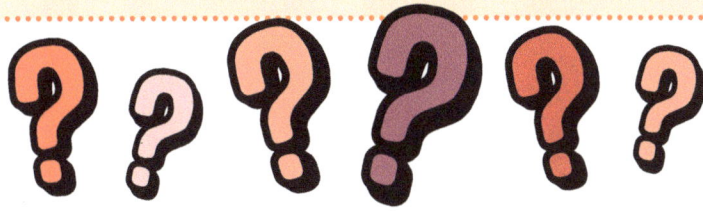

WHERE IS WHAT IN YOUR BODY?

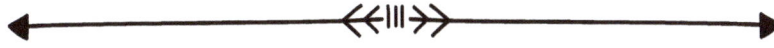

Skin is our biggest organ. Label other major parts.
Happy Heart Healthy Choices help keep everything happy.

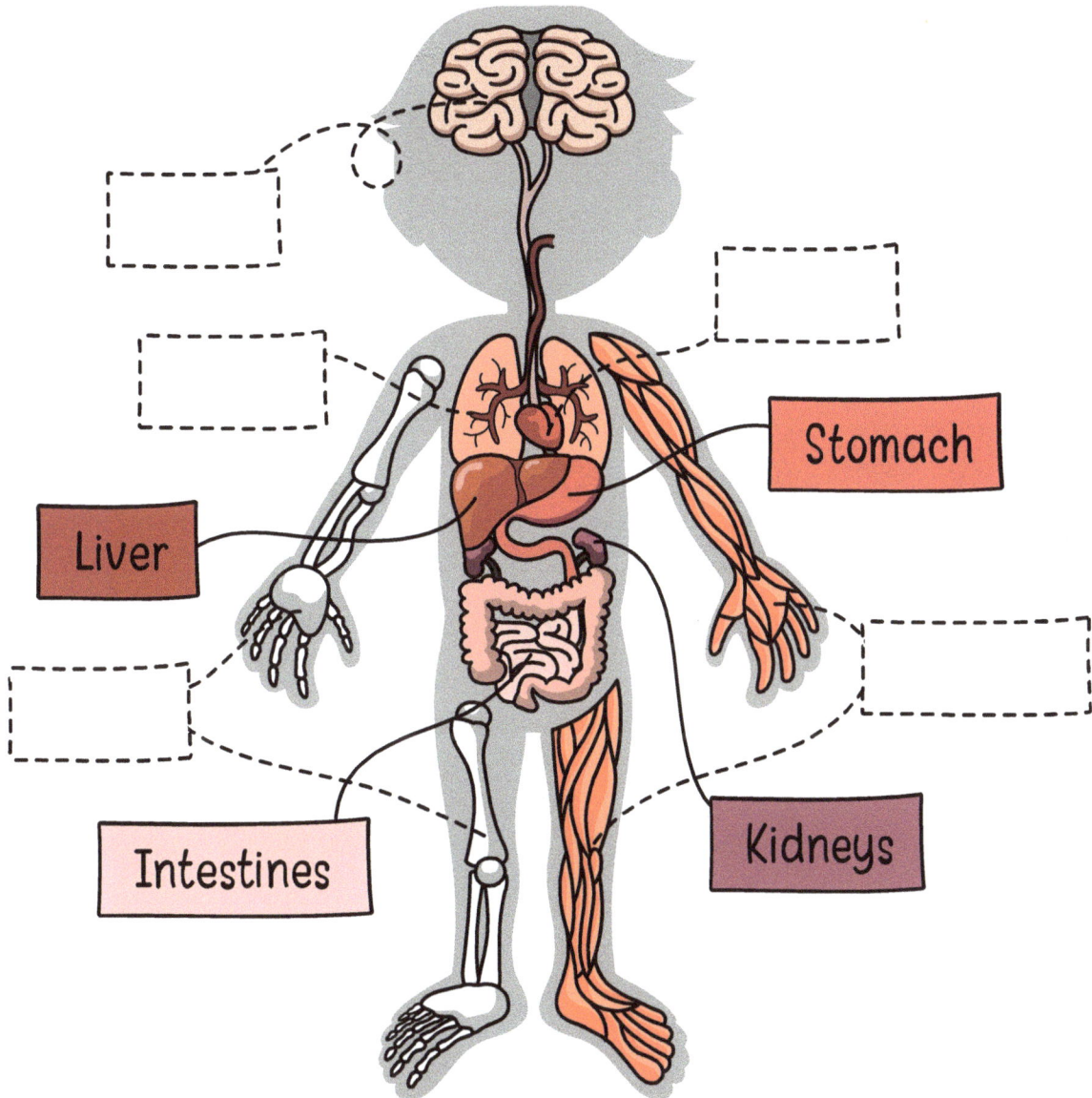

Stomach

Liver

Intestines

Kidneys

Muscles   Lungs   Bones   Brain   Heart

UNDERSTANDING THE DIFFERENCE

6-12-year-olds need between 1600 to 2200 food points (calories) each day to grow and develop. This amount is based on one's body type, metabolism genetics, physical activity and even the weather.

Understanding food points (calories) lets you make **Happy Healthy Heart Smart** choices. Too many **Sad Heart** points puts the body out of balance.

100 Happy Healthy Heart snack food point portions:

100 Sad Heart snack food point portions:

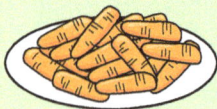 1 Orange **VS.** 1/3 Donut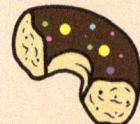

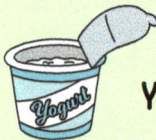 25 Baby Carrots **VS.** 9 Regular Chips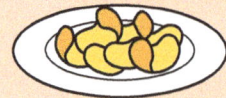

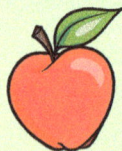 1/2 cup Yogurt Dip **VS.** 1 Tablespoon Ranch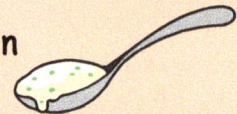

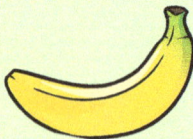 1 Apple **VS.** 1 Halloween Sized Candy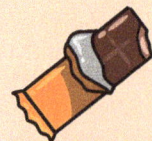

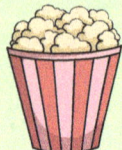 1 Whole Medium Banana **VS.** 1/2 Mega Stuffed Oreo

4 Cups Of Air Popped Popcorn **VS.** 10 Fast Food French Fries + 1 Ketchup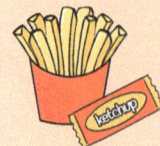

CHECK IT OUT!

FRUIT FRACTIONS

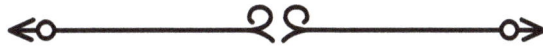

Color in the fiber, antioxidant, vitamin and mineral SUPER ME GRR8 fruits.

Numerator: Write the amount of each kind of fruit in their yellow box.
Denominator: Write the total number of all fruit in the blue boxes.

Can the numerator and denominator be divided by the same number?
Reduce each fraction to lowest terms.

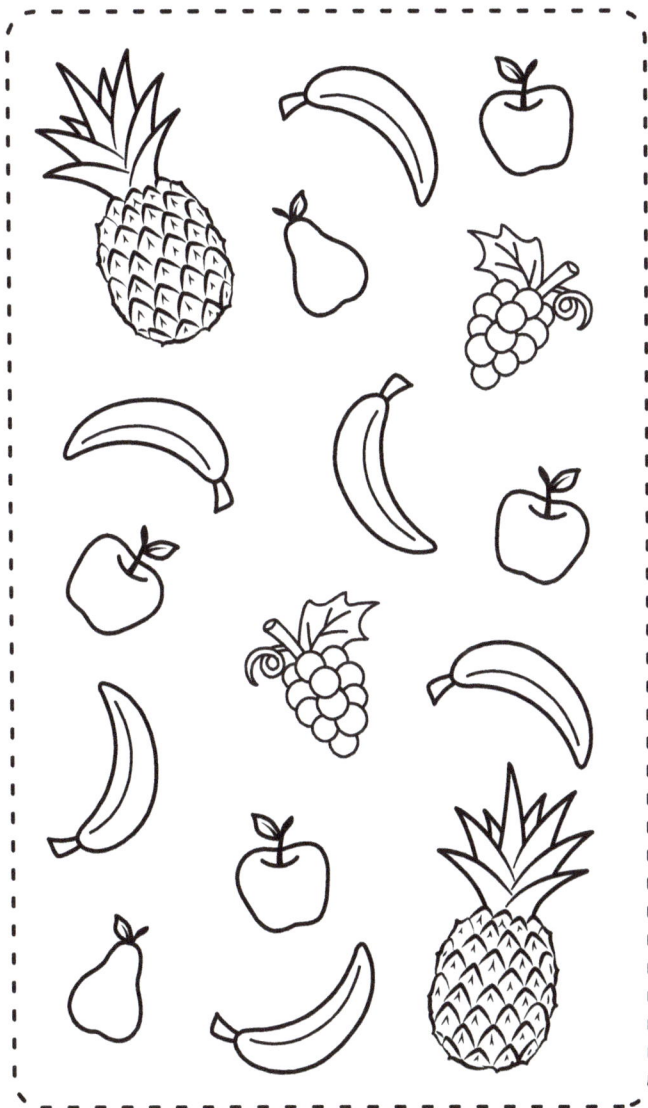

$$\frac{4}{16} \div \frac{4}{4} = \frac{1}{4}$$

READY, SET, OFF TO SCHOOL WE GO

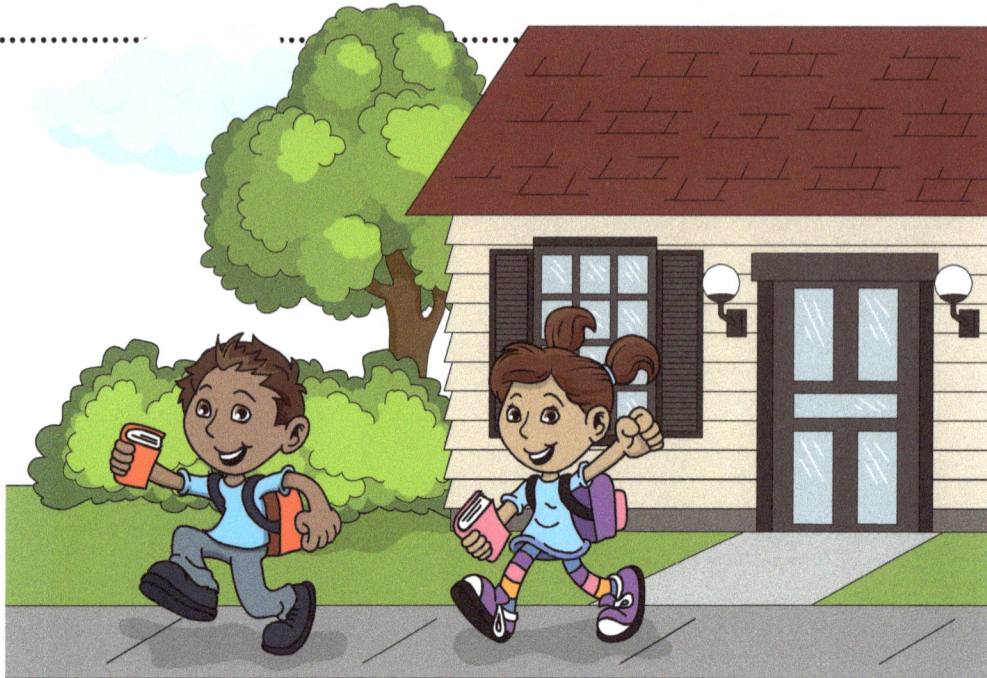

The breakfast table is cleared. Our lunches are made. School and lunch bags are by the door. We hop/skip into the bathroom to brush and floss teeth. We put a pea-sized amount of toothpaste on our brushes.

We set the timer for two minutes for "exer-brush". We do a mini workout as we gently brush our teeth, gums and tongue!

We twist our bodies, squat, balance on tip toes or swing our legs. Mom says every bit of movement helps keep our blood pumping!

Save water and go mobile:
Always turn off the water while you brush your teeth. This saves lots of wonderful clean drinking water! Use your saliva or put some water in a cup.
Since your mouth isn't bubbling, you can stretch while you brush! Turn on the water to rinse. **Win-Win- Win:** Teeth brushed, extra exercise and planet saved!

THINK ABOUT IT!

CHECK IT OUT!

27

After we spit and rinse, it is time to floss carefully between our teeth. It is like playing "Hide and Go Seek" with my food. I like to look at my string to see what I can catch. Sometimes, tiny bits of food hide between my teeth. If they hide better than I seek, germs start to grow.

Germs rot teeth and make nice pink gums sick. Healthy gums keep teeth from falling out!

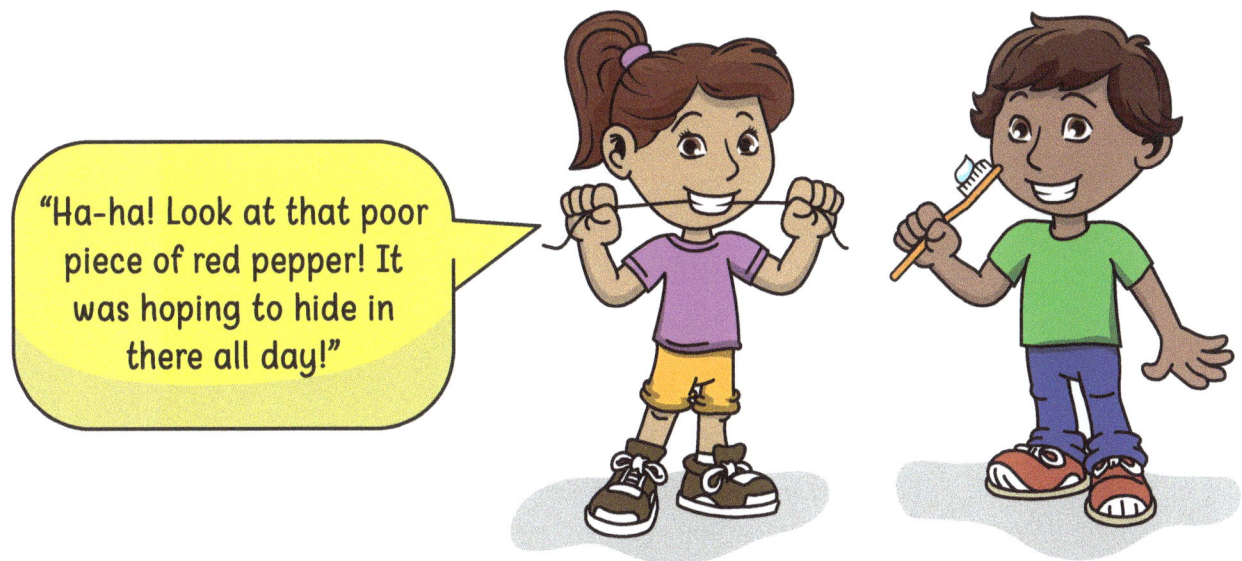

"Ha-ha! Look at that poor piece of red pepper! It was hoping to hide in there all day!"

Once our teeth are clean, we go into the big room for our morning silly-giggly-wiggly time. Each morning, we dance, hop, hula-hoop, jump, sing and giggle.

After 10 minutes of going crazy, we fall on the floor laughing, totally exhausted, yet full of energy.

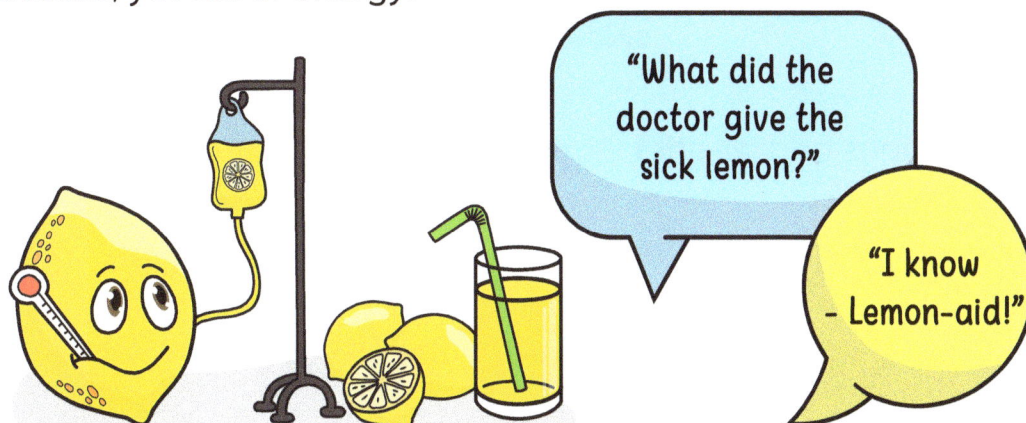

"What did the doctor give the sick lemon?"

"I know - Lemon-aid!"

CHECK IT OUT!

Our family starts every day with a glass of water and a great breakfast to fuel our metabolism, mind and body.

We make **Happy Healthy Heart** breakfasts and lunches that cost less than a can of soda.

A little crazy dancing gets our hearts pumping and causes a whole lot of laughing.

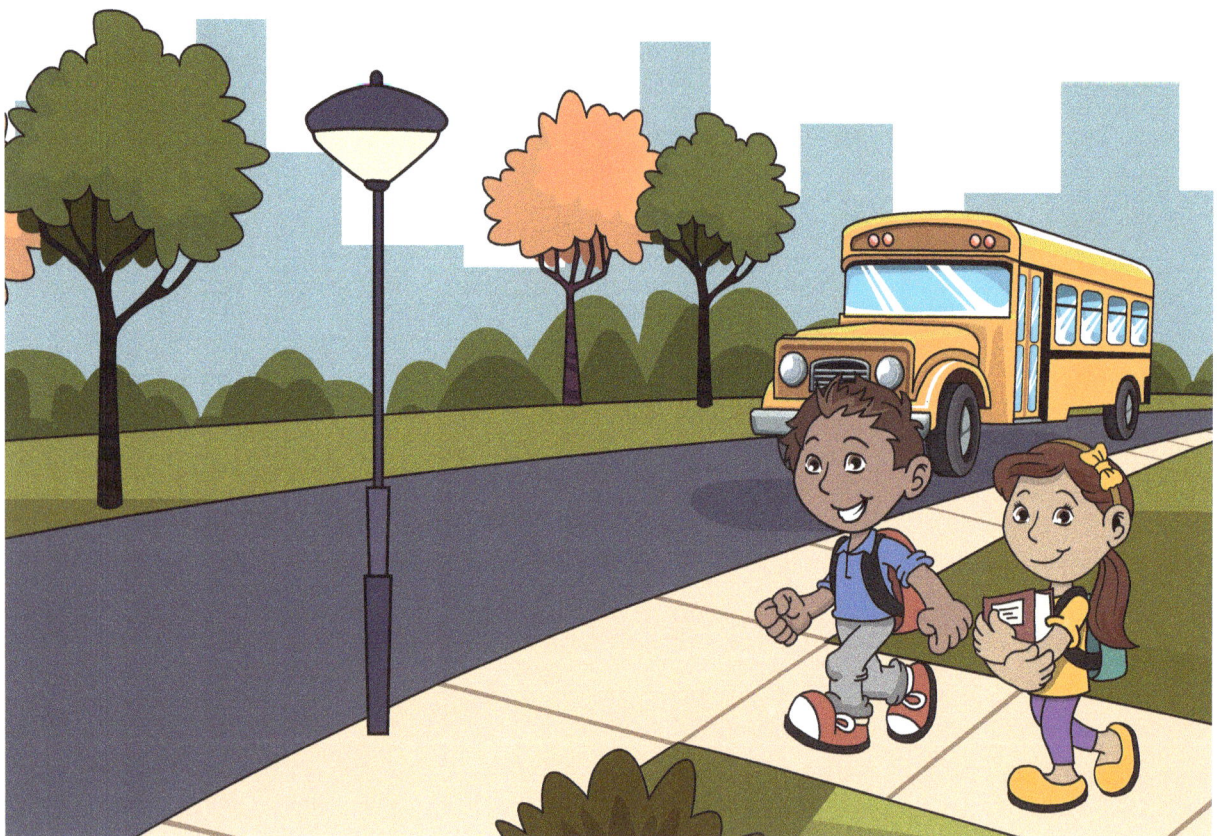

We grab our bags and go out to catch the bus.

As the bus comes closer, Mom kisses us. *"Have a great day. Give your best. Learn something new. Remember, always be kind."*

MOVING AND GROOVING

Imagine your cousins are coming for a visit from another country. They don't speak English. They want to teach friends back home an exercise they learned.

Draw the different steps of your favorite exercise for them to take home. Number each step.

My .... Exercise

CHECK IT OUT!

WHY IS A HEALTHY HAPPY HEART IMPORTANT?

The heart is a huge pump. It pushes blood to cells in every corner of the body through super highways called arteries*. Our cells need the nutrient* and oxygen (O2)-packed blood to keep us alive.

Cells gobble up the yummy nutrients and O2 and send them back through veins* filled with carbon dioxide (CO2).

Now the heart and lungs work together as a recycling factory. CO2 and other "trash"-filled blood are turned back to clean healthy O2-rich blood. At a speed of about 3 feet per second, in less than 60 seconds, new blood is pumped to every cell.

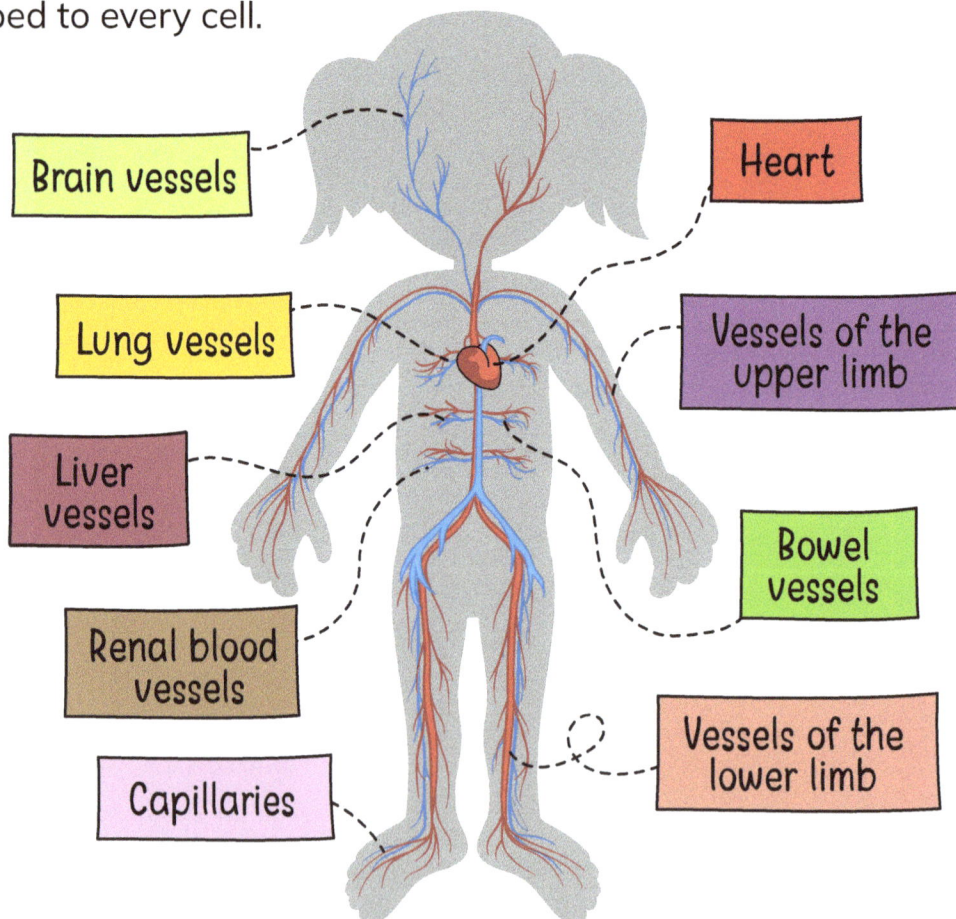

Brain vessels

Heart

Lung vessels

Vessels of the upper limb

Liver vessels

Renal blood vessels

Bowel vessels

Capillaries

Vessels of the lower limb

*(**ART**-er-ee) The little tubes that deliver blood to the body.
(**NEW**-tree-ant) Something that boosts growth, improves energy and supports life.
(vane) Any tube that return blood to the heart.

CHECK
IT OUT!

The heart cleans almost three bathtubs full of blood a day
A happy healthy heart = more oxygen pumped into my blood.
More oxygen in my blood fuels my brain = smarter, healthier me!

The more salt we eat the harder the kidneys and bladder work.
This can cause blood pressure problems which are very dangerous for the heart.

DID YOU KNOW?

Your pulse or the "Lub-Dub" sound you hear is your heart valves shutting.

Find your pulse on the side of your neck or the inside of your wrist, just below your thumb. Press lightly where you see a large artery below your skin. The small beat you feel is your pulse.

Use a clock with seconds or the stopwatch on a cell phone to count the number of beats you feel in 1 minute. This is your resting heart rate.

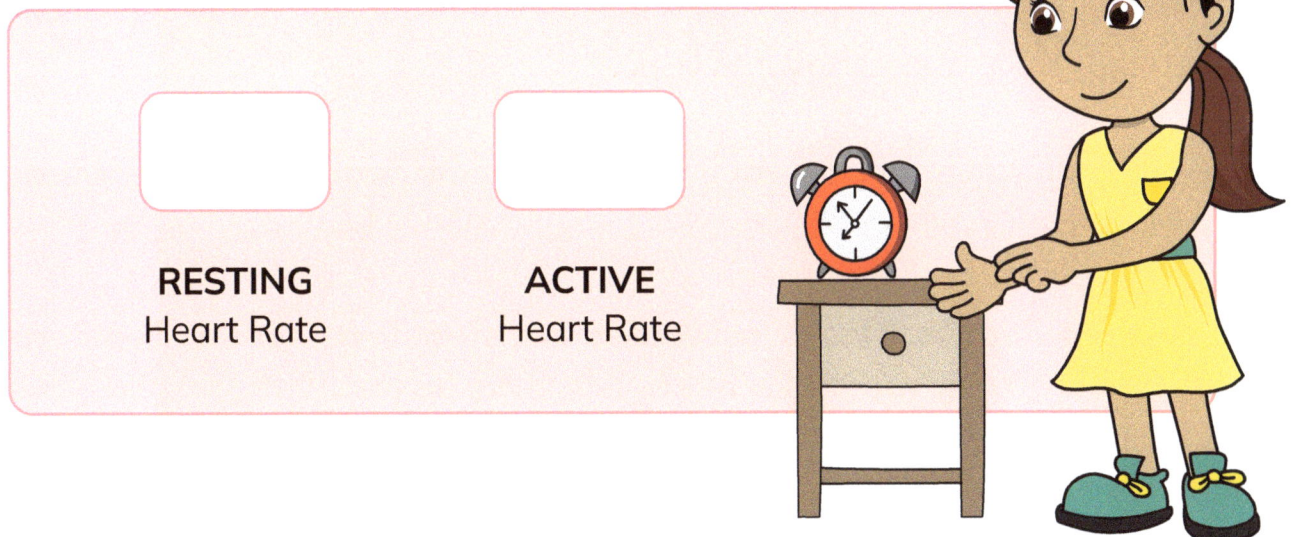

RESTING
Heart Rate

ACTIVE
Heart Rate

Now, jump up and down, run, or do jumping jacks for one minute. Recount your pulse. This is your active pulse. Did it change? Why?

CHECK IT OUT!

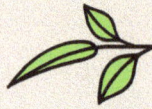

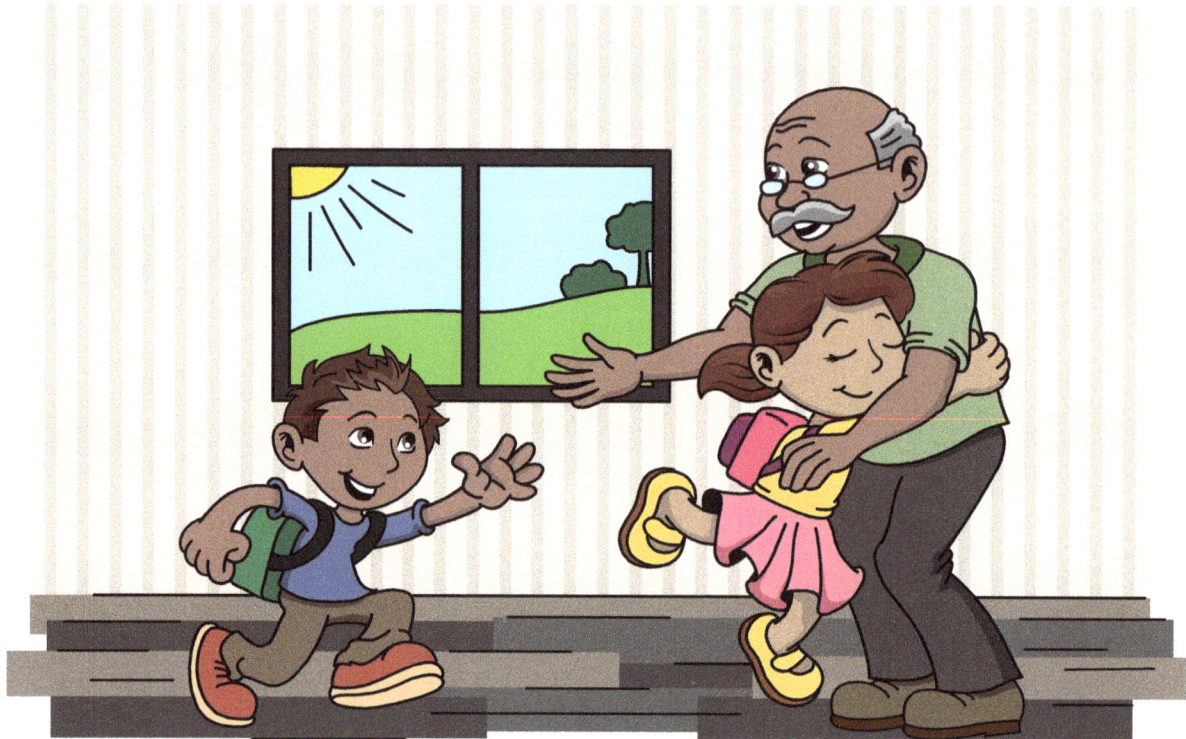

"*Hi, Grandpa. We're home!*" we sing, as we run in the door. "*How was your day?*" we ask our favorite G-pa.

G-pa laughs, "*Let me see you. This is my favorite day. Those sweet smiles are my medicine!*" He hugs both of us tightly in his big strong arms.

"*I made a little snack for us to nibble before we go to the garden. You know how I love to play with food,*" he says. "*Hip hop to the bathroom and wash your hands. Turn off the water. Count to 20 while you rub and bubble.*"

We actually hop off to wash our hands. When Grandpa says, "hop", he means it!

"What do you suppose G-pa made us this time?" I ask.

BB shakes his head. With G-pa, it is always a surprise.

Hands washed, we skip back to the kitchen and look at the table.

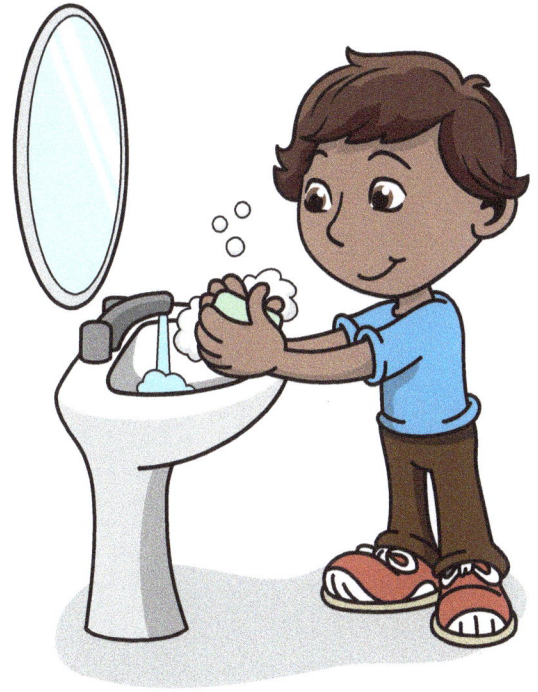

"What is the hardest part of being an octopus?"

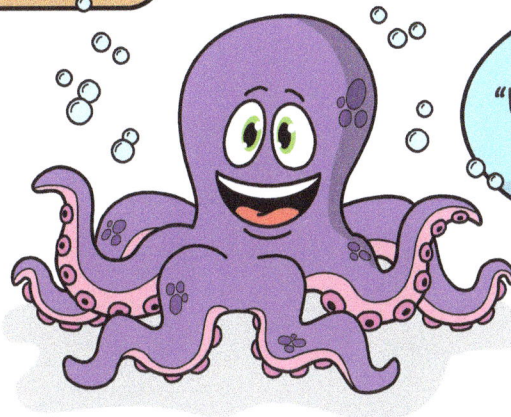

"Washing your hands before eating!"

"Peanut butter scary faces! That's what happens to your beautiful smiles if you don't eat right and take good care of your teeth." He laughs, pointing to the faces with black raisin teeth.

We all laugh as we gobble up the raisin smiles, peanut butter faces, grape eyes, celery noses, banana hair and apple ears.

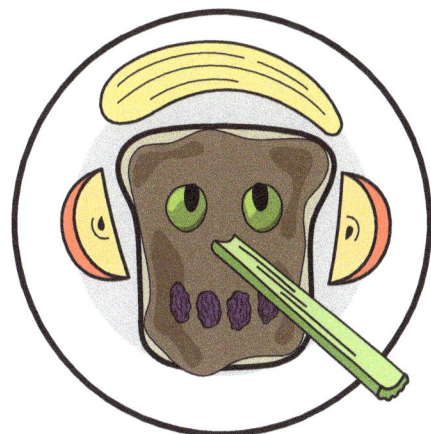

SUPER ME REVOLUTION CHALLENGE

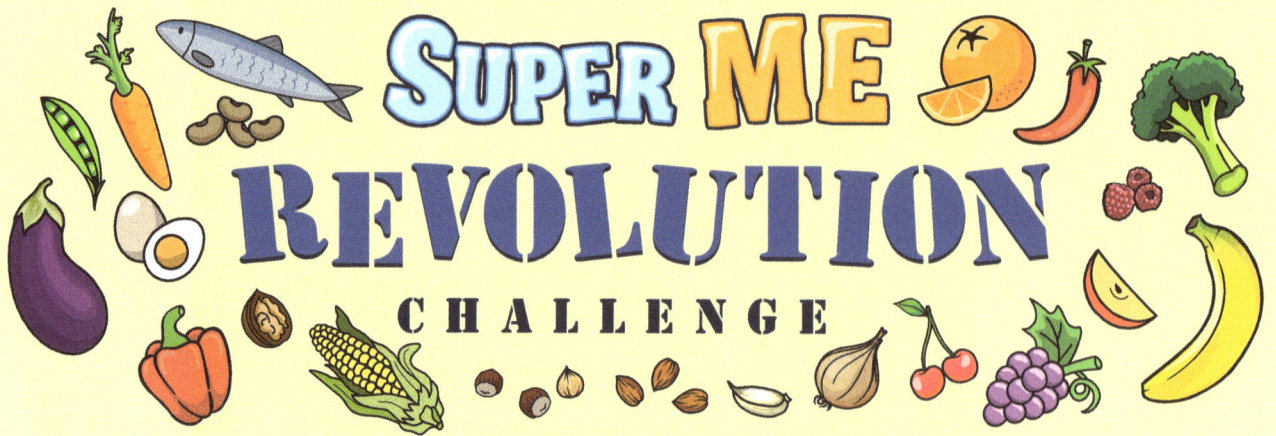

"I am so excited to hear about all the things you learned in school today," G-pa says, as we sit around the table.

I jump right in. "Our whole school signed up for the Super Me Revolution Challenge. Our principal says learning to keep our bodies and minds healthy is as important as all our other classes."

"Kids who eat kid-size **Happy Healthy Heart** foods and exercise 40 minutes a day usually do better in school. Plus, they are more likely to learn a trade or go to college.

We all agreed to become 'Health Champions' and share what we learn with our families. Did you know **Every Bite Matters?** Even the smallest **Happy Healthy Heart** changes are GRRR8."

"We promised to drink more water, get our hearts pumping, understand kid-size portions, and learn how to prepare **Happy Healthy Heart** foods."

"We talked about Made@Home vs. PreMade food. Made@Home food means we know exactly what we are eating, because we made it! Premade food is expensive and tricks us into wanting more because of the fat, sugar, and salt hiding inside. Plus, we think a prepared serving is a normal portion, so we gobble it all up. It is usually way too big for kids."

CHECK IT OUT!

35

"Learn tricks to eat kid-sized portions is super important. The EJ 1/2 Trick ('Eat-Just-Half') helps when eating prepared foods. Sometimes portions are so big. EJ 1/4 is a better trick!" I say laughing.

"Our homework is to make one Make@Home food each night. We use healthy websites for ideas like SuperMe!, MyPlate.Org, Cooking With Kids, Cooking Up Change, HealthyChildren.Org, or Jamie Oliver's Kids Cooking.

We find seven recipes our family will like, watch how-to videos, write down directions and what we will need. On the weekend, we help shop.

"We learn to read labels for healthier choices. Many healthy Make@Home Happy Heart foods like beans, eggs, oats, quinoa and frozen veggies are easy to make. They give us lots more healthy food for our money, too."

"Most of the kids in my class have never helped in the kitchen. They were scared at first, but there are lots of cooking videos online to help," I explain.

"Another part of our challenge is to write down everything we eat and drink each day. We keep a log of the 'Make@Home Happy Heart Foods' and 'Premade Foods' we eat. Keeping logs lets us see patterns in our choices," I explain.

KNOW WHAT YOU EAT!

My Heart Smart Food /Pre-Made Food Log

If you can say all the ingredients in your food choice, chances are it fits in the **Heart Smart** side.

MAKE@HOME HEART SMART FOOD	PREMADE FOOD			

YOU BE THE JUDGE!

Pick a new fruit, vegetable or **Happy Healthy Heart** recipe to try. After tasting, rate it on how it looks, smells, tastes and how it feels in your mouth. Give it a score with 5 being the best. For more fun, play this game with your friends or people in your family. Take it to the next level and compare 3 new foods.

Draw it here

Visual Appeal

1 2 3 4 5

Smell

1 2 3 4 5

Taste

1 2 3 4 5

Texture

1 2 3 4 5

Total score: ....

The result is:

☐ I think I might need a few more tries to get used to it.

☐ I will eat it again, soon. I am glad I tried it.

☐ It is GRRR8! I love it! I am glad I tried it.

CHECK IT OUT!

THE ATTACK OF THE SUGAR MONSTER

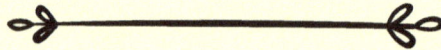

Scientists discovered that every time we eat something with sugar, it tricks our brain to want more sugar. The more sugar we eat or drink, the more sugar our brain demands! Too much sugar rots our teeth and causes really big health problems. Trying to cut back on too much sugar in our daily intake is really hard. Using substitute sugars can cause other problems because our brain still wants lots of sweet things.

Doctors say it is as hard to fight the Sugar Monster as trying to quit smoking. The more Big Bully Sugar Monster controls our choices, the harder it is to get free. It growls for more when we try to eat less. This is really hard because sugar is hiding everywhere - in mayonnaise, bread, breakfast cereal, ketchup, pizza, or even fries.

Enjoy a little sugar in ice cream, cake or candy, not hiding in our meals.

DID YOU KNOW?

Factories put sugar, fat and salt into almost everything. This combination tricks our brain and our taste buds to always want more. Our brain tells us to buy that product because we think it is the best, even though we may know it is not.

THINK ABOUT IT!

Ranch dressing is mostly oil, sugar and salt. Is eating a bowl of ranch a good or bad idea for your heart?

Circle the correct answer. **GOOD** 👍 **BAD** 👎

VALUE: RANCH DRESSING VS. ICE CREAM

¼ cup of ranch dressing = 230 calories or food points.

½ cup of ice cream = 115 calories or food points.

1 cup	—	250
3/4	—	200
1/2	—	150
1/4	—	100

cup   food points

1 cup	—	250
3/4	—	200
1/2	—	150
1/4	—	100

cup   food points

Ranch Dressing Measuring Cup

- Draw a line to mark ¼ cup.
- Draw a line to mark the number of food points per serving.
- Color each side to the line marks with a different color.

Ice Cream Measuring Cup

- Draw a line to show 1/2 cup.
- Draw a line to mark the number of food points.
- Color each side to the line marks with a different color.

Both of these are full of fat and sugar.

Which gives you more value for your food points?   Ice Cream / Ranch

Which makes your heart happier: a snack of plain carrots or carrots dipped in ranch dressing?   With / Without

Which sugar and fat points taste better? Why?   Ice Cream / Ranch

_____

_____

THINK ABOUT IT!

SODA VS. WATER — WHAT'S THE BIG DIFFERENCE?

The National Heart Association says kids need **6** teaspoons (tsp.) of sugar a day. This includes sugars found in fruit and milk.

With all the hidden sugars in premade food and soda, kids usually have about **21** teaspoons a day.

This adds up to about **30 gallons** each year. That is more than fills a big bathtub.

SODA CAN

Serving Size 1 can (12 fl oz)	
Serving Per Container 1	

Amount Per Serving	
Calories 150	

	% Daily Values*
Total Fat 0g	0%
Saturated Fat 0g	
Trans Fat 0g	
Cholesterol 0mg	0%
Sodium 45mg	2%
Total Carbohydrate 40g	13%
Dietary Fiber 0g	
Sugars 40g	
Protein 0g	0%

Ingredients:

Carbonated Water, High Fructose Corn Syrup, Caramel Color, Phosphoric Acid, Natural Flavors, Caffeine

---

How many tsp. of sugar should a child have in one year?

[   ] tsp. per week **× 48** weeks per year = [   ] tsp. (round up or down)

How much is that in pounds?

[   ] tsp. **/60** = [   ] lbs. (round up or down)

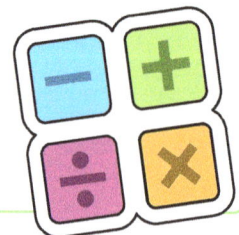

> 60 tsp = 1 pound (lbs)

How many tsp. of sugar do many children usually have in one year?

[   ] tsp. per week **× 48** weeks per year = [   ] tsp. (round up or down)

How much is that in pounds?

[   ] tsp. **/60** = [   ] lbs. (round up or down)

WOW — IT ADDS UP FAST!

Your cousin drinks one can of soda every day.
How much sugar will he drink in one year?

How many grams of sugar is in one 12 ounce (oz.) can of soda? [ ] g.

What is that equal to in teaspoons (tsp.)?

[ ] g. ÷ 4 = [ ] tsp. in one 12 oz. can.

> **4 grams of sugar = 1 teaspoon (tsp.)**

How many tsp. of sugar will he drink in one year?

[ ] tsp. per week **x 48** weeks per year = [ ] tsp. (round up or down)

How much is that in pounds?

[ ] tsp. ÷ **60** = [ ] lbs. (round up or down)

> **60 tsp. = 1 pound (lbs.)**

One gallon of water weighs about 3 pounds.
How many bottles would it take to fill in the sugar?

[ ] lbs. ÷ **3** = [ ] bottles

> Pounds of sugar a child should have in one year: [ ]

> Pounds of sugar from one can of soda each day: [ ]

TRICK

Break down the 12 into 10 + 2.
First multiply by 10 (That's easy: Add a zero!)
Then multiply again by 2.
Now, add the two sums together.

> **Example:**
> $32 \times 12 \nearrow^{10+2}$
> $32 \times 10 + 32 \times 2$
> $320 + 64$
> $= 384$

CHECK IT OUT!

READ THE SMALL PRINT
AND THE BIG WORDS EXPERIMENT

The label on the back of every food item is like a report card. It helps us make **Happy Healthy Heart** Smart choices.

It tells how many adult servings are in one container and how many calories (food points) are in each serving.

It lists all the ingredients. The ingredient that makes up the most of the food is listed first.

The last ingredient is the smallest amount. Sweeteners near the top means lots of hidden sugar points.

The amount of things an adult needs each day like vitamins, minerals, protein and fiber are listed, too. Kids, of course, need different amounts.

Circle all the words for 'sweetener' listed in the label.

MARSHMALLOW BAG

| Serving Size 12 | |
| Serving Per Container 4 (29 g.) | |

Amount Per Serving	
Calories 100	
	% Daily Values*
Total Fat 0g	0%
Sodium 30mg	1%
Total Carbohydrate 9g	34%
Sugars 17g	
Protein Less than 1g	0%

Not a significant source of Calories from Fat, Saturated Fat, Trans Fat, Cholesterol, Dietary Fiber, Vitamin A, Vitamin C, Calcium and Iron.

*Percent Daily Values are based on a 2,000 calorie diet.

Ingredients: Corn Syrup, Sugar, Dextrose, Modified Cornstarch, Water, Contains Less Than 2% Of Gelatin, Tetrasodium, pyrophosphate (whipping aid), natural and artificial flavor, Blue 1.

DID YOU KNOW?

Different names for sweeteners:
Agave, brown sugar, corn sweetener, corn syrup, carbitol, coconut sugar, concentrated fruit juice, date sugar, dextrose, diglycerides, disaccharides, erythritol, evaporated cane juice, erythritol, Florida crystals, fructooligosaccharides, fructose, galactose, glucitol, glucosamine, glucose, hexitol, inversol, high-fructose corn syrup, honey, isomalt, lactose, malted barley, maltose, malt syrup, malts, maple syrup, molasses, maltodextrin, mannitol, nectars, pentose, raisin syrup, raw sugar, ribose, rice malt, rice syrup, rice syrup solids, sorbitol, sorghum, starch, stavia, sucrose, sucanat, sugar, xylitol and xylose.

CHECK IT OUT!

My friend is trying to make healthy choices.
The bag says marshmallows are fat-free. Can she eat all she wants?

HYPOTHESIS

Eating a small bag of fat-free marshmallows each day is a wise choice for a healthy lifestyle.

YES   **NO**

(Circle which you <u>think</u> is correct.)

RESEARCH

How many servings are in one bag?

How many food points (calories) are in one serving?

Number of food points (calories) are in one bag of marshmallows?

Most children should eat between 1400 and 2200 food points (calories) each day. How many daily food points (calories) are left after eating the bag of fat-free marshmallows?

[ ] −	[ ] =	[ ]
Number of servings in one bag	Food Points/Calories per serving	Food Points/ Calories per bag

She used [ ] food points on marshmallows. How much protein, which her body needs each day for her muscles, bones, skin and blood has she eaten?

How much fiber for a clean digestive system has she eaten?

What is the main ingredient in marshmallows?

....

What is the second most used ingredient?

....

Do you think she is spending her daily food points wisely?

....

CONCLUSION

Eating a small bag of fat free marshmallows each day is a wise choice for a healthy lifestyle.

YES   **NO**

(Circle which you <u>know</u> is correct, based on your research.)

"IF YOU HAVE A GARDEN AND A LIBRARY,
YOU HAVE EVERYTHING YOU NEED."

- Marcus Tullius Cicero

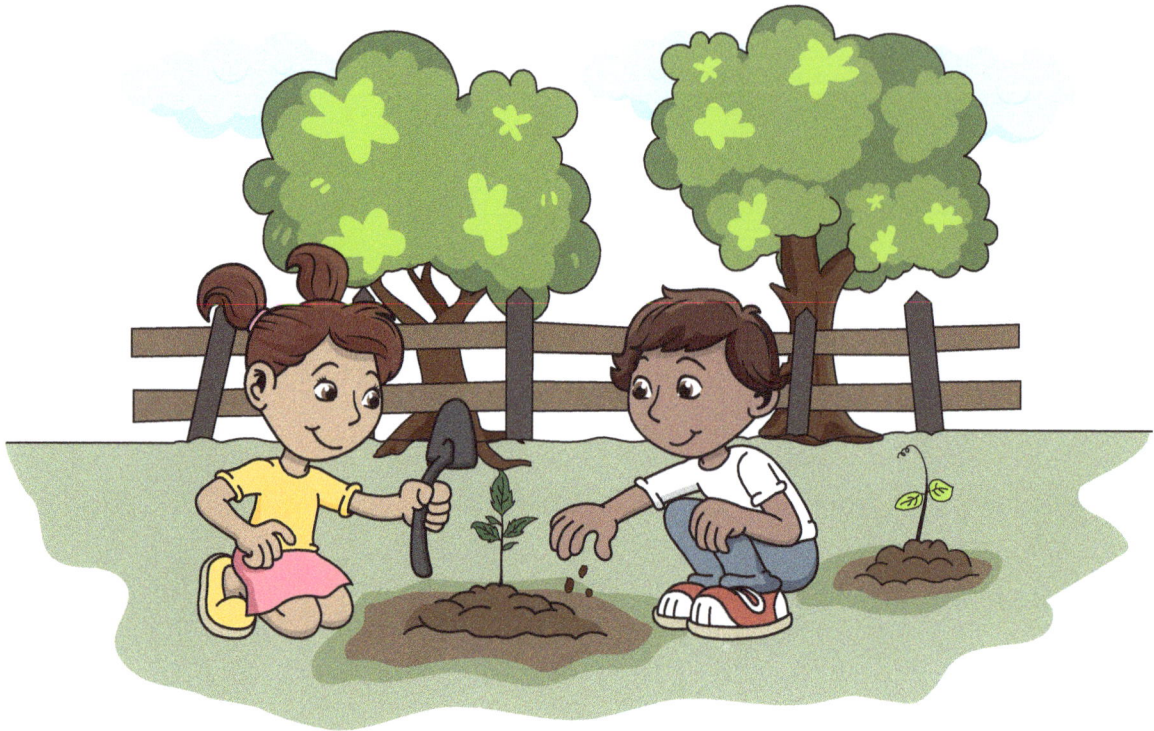

A few years ago, our school decided to start a garden. Lots of people helped make our dream come true.

Neighbors gave us seeds and small plants. People who grew up farming, taught us how to plan and prepare the beds. Our library and *The Edible Schoolyard Project* had lots of ideas. Parents helped build boxes for our planter beds. We put in gravel paths to help with drainage. Strangers helped build our wonderful shed and the big, beautiful fence that surrounds our garden, keeping the bunnies out and everything safe.

We are so proud of the magic garden our community helped build and all the new friends we made.

We grow lots of yummy healthy fruits, vegetables, herbs and even flowers we eat! We eat our fresh from the ground! Sometimes, it takes only seconds from plant-to-mouth before we gobble them up!

Everything tastes **GRRR8** because we only harvest when the produce is ripe. Commercial growers must pick everything much earlier because their produce travels for days and days by trucks, trains, planes and sometimes even boats before arriving in the stores.

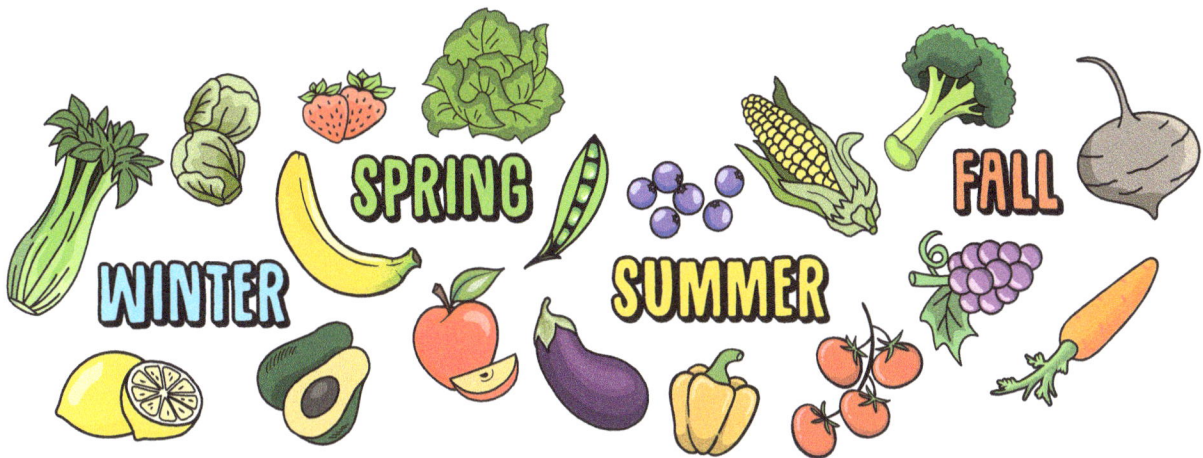

WINTER SPRING SUMMER FALL

We keep growing, even in the winter!

Each fall, we grow "cold weather" plants like spinach, salad greens, cabbage, mint, parsley, rosemary, chives and scallions.

Root veggies (potatoes, turnips, carrots, radishes, and onions) actually love the cold. Winter weather makes them even sweeter.

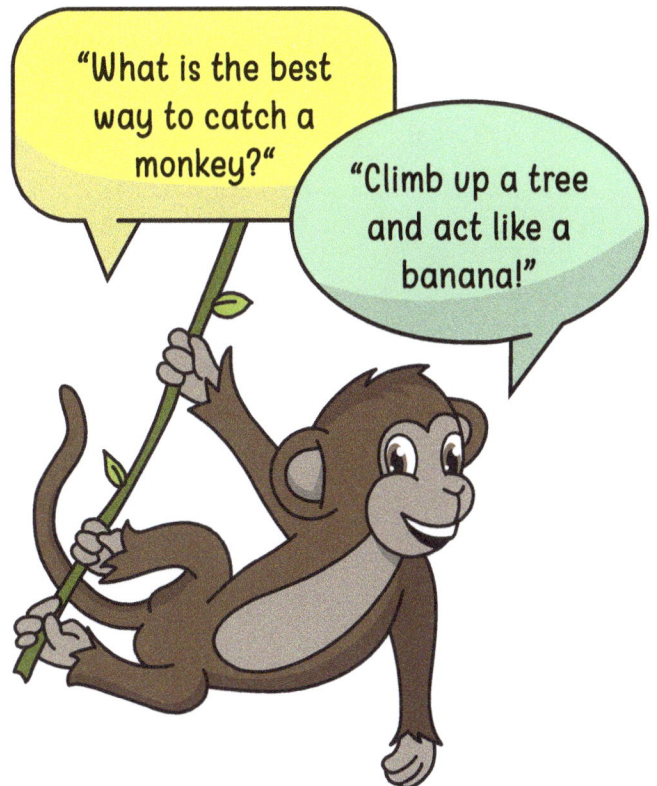

"What is the best way to catch a monkey?"

"Climb up a tree and act like a banana!"

Towards the end of winter, we start growing our seeds indoors. It is so exciting to see tiny baby leaves start to peek out from the soil.

In springtime, when the nights are warmer, we plant our babies in the beds outside. Every two weeks, we start 'Crazy Yummy Carrot' seeds. This keeps us munching all through the seasons.

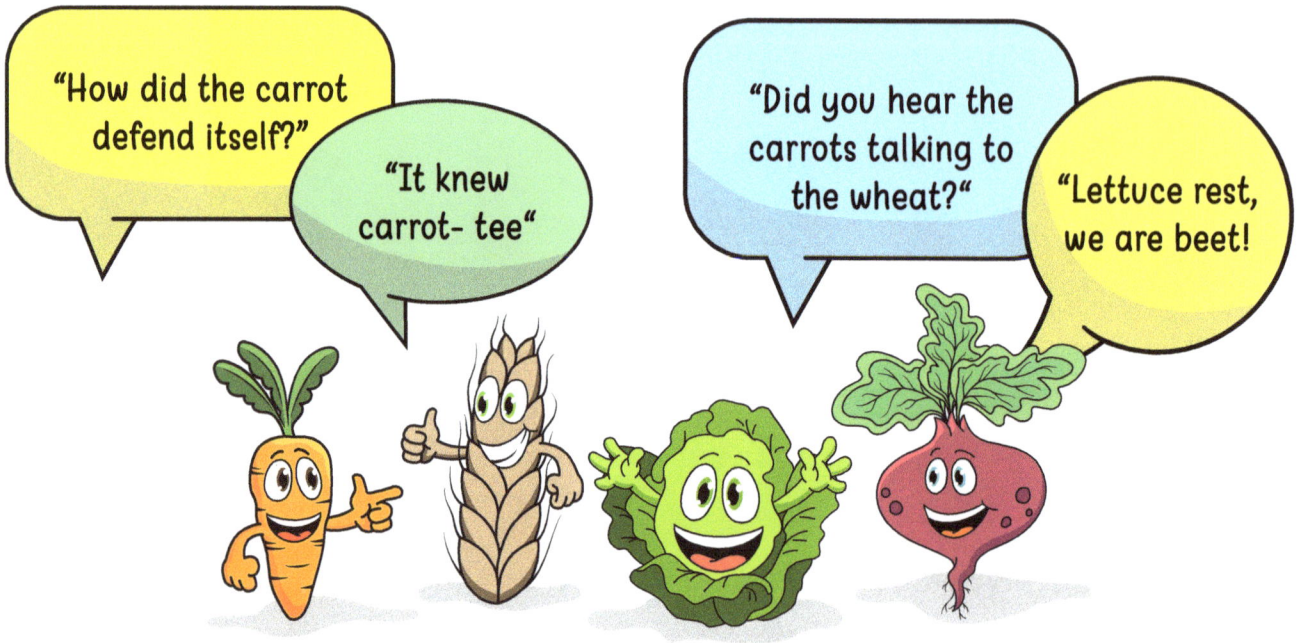

"How did the carrot defend itself?"

"It knew carrot- tee"

"Did you hear the carrots talking to the wheat?"

"Lettuce rest, we are beet!

Marcus Tualius Cicero was a Roman philosopher*, politician, lawyer, and public speaker. He was born in 106 BCE and died in 43 BCE. His writings helped inspire the founding of the United States almost 1800 years after he lived.

What do you think he meant when he said, "If you have a garden and a library, you have everything you need"?

....

....

....

CHECK IT OUT!

(fi-**LOSS**-ah-fur) Someone who thinks about the meaning of things.
Philosophy (fi-**LOSS**-ah-fee) is the love or study of wisdom. It asks questions like: Are people mostly good or evil? What is more important, doing things right or doing the right thing? What is happiness? What is love? Do animals have feelings?

HELP DESIGN OUR GARDEN BEDS

Our vegetable garden is ready to plant. The Three Sisters: pumpkins, corn and beans always go together. (p. 101) Watermelons need extra space, too. Celery is a must because we eat everything- roots, leaves, stalks, seeds, even the flowers. Peas climb on fences.

0 → 1 → 2 → 3 feet

Draw lines for this year's garden design. Label each section with a drawing so we know what and where to plant.

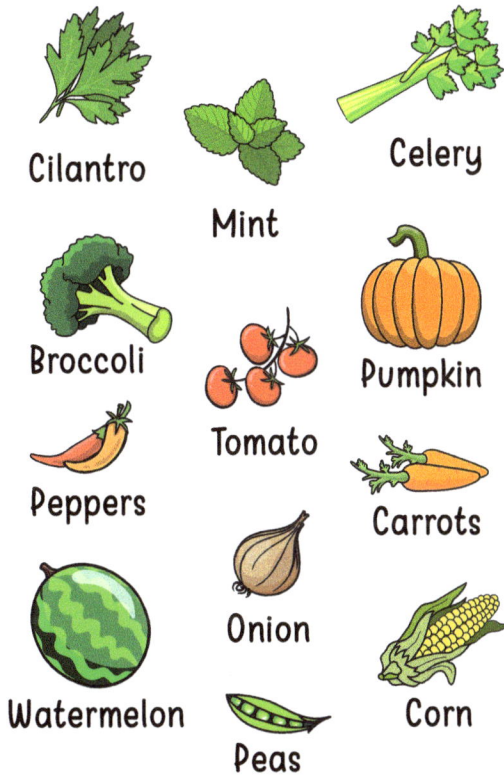

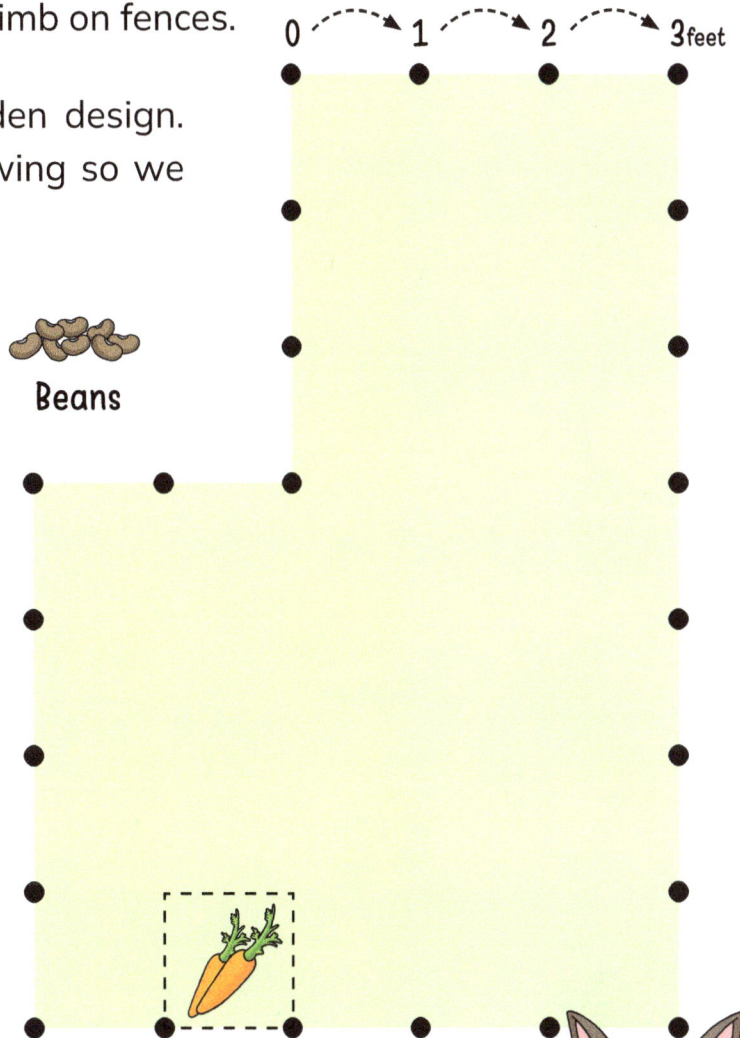

Cilantro

Mint

Celery

Beans

Broccoli

Tomato

Pumpkin

Peppers

Carrots

Watermelon

Onion

Corn

Peas

We need a fence to keep out the rabbits. Help us calculate the perimeter. Each dot is a fence post = one foot apart.

3 + ⬚ + ⬚ + ⬚ + ⬚ + ⬚ = ⬚ feet

TRICK Find the perimeter by adding together the lengths of all the sides.

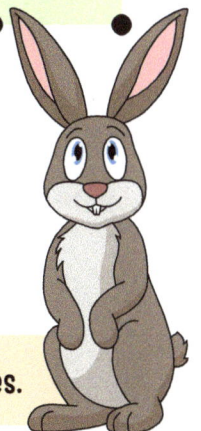

WHAT PART OF THE PLANT DO WE EAT?

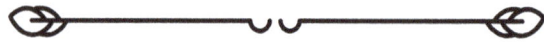

Is it a Fruit? Is it a Vegetable?

Botanists* say fruits have seeds. Vegetables are roots, stems, leaves and even flower buds. Cooks say if it is sweet, it is a fruit. This is why many fruits like tomato, avocado, cucumber and peas switch between the groups.

Connect the pictures to the words that best describe the part we eat. Some belong to more than one group. For example, every part of celery is edible, so it belongs to ALL groups!

CARROT

ONION

PUMPKIN

CELERY

BROCCOLI

CORN

BEANS

TOMATO

LEMON

FRUIT

STEM

SEED

LEAF

ROOT/TUBER

APPLE

BANANA

GREEN BEANS

POTATO

RICE

JICAMA

GRAPES

STRAWBERRY

PINEAPPLE

LETTUCE

*(**BAWT**-an-ist) a person who studies plants.

CHECK IT OUT!

With a ruler, connect vegetables to vegetables and fruits to fruits.
Use different colors to create your very own artwork.

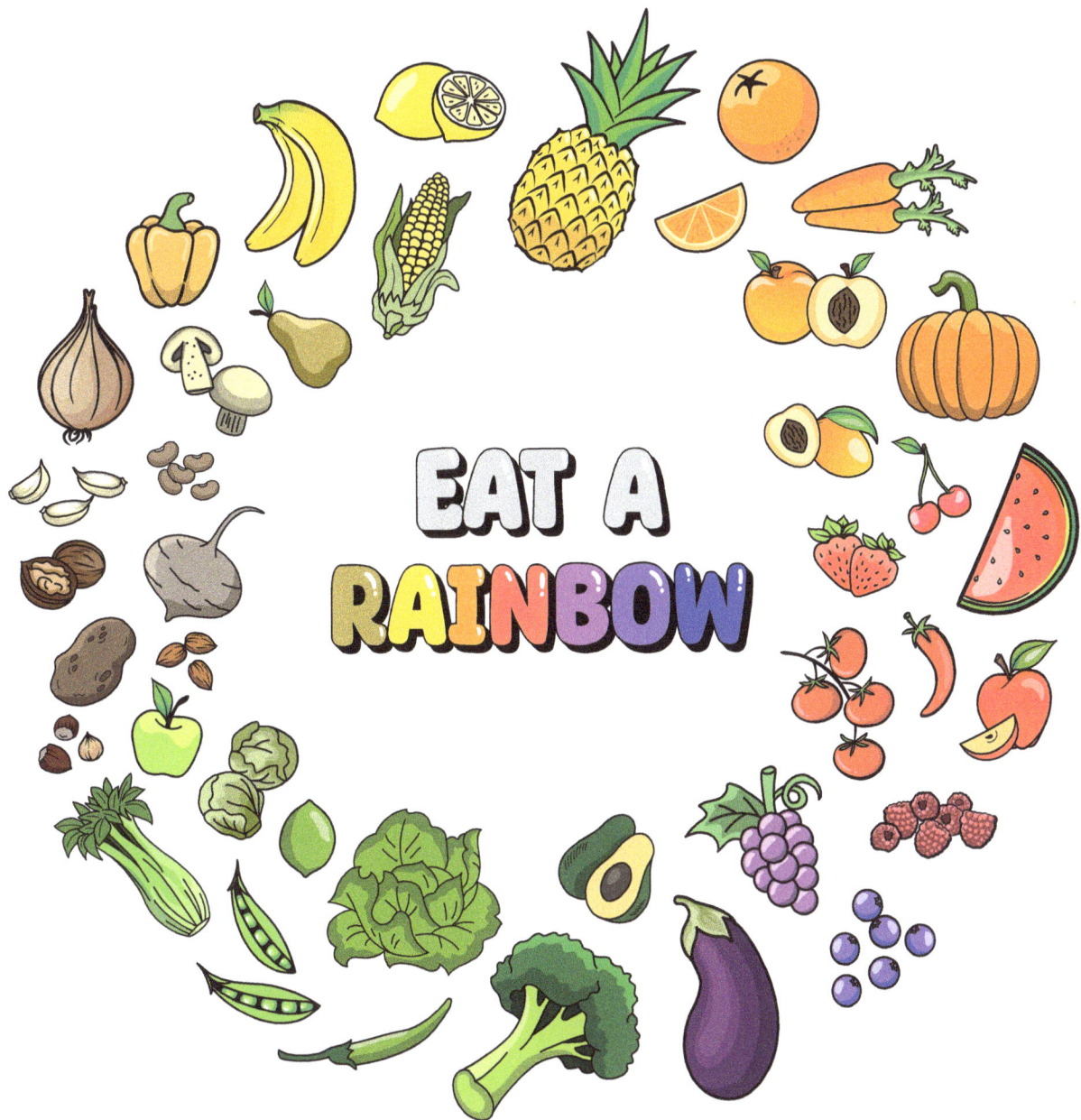

EAT A
RAINBOW

Vitamin C helps fight diseases, keeps us from getting sick, protects our cells, and heals our wounds. Our bodies use Vitamin C to absorb other vitamins, as well.

Great sources of Vitamin C are pineapple, broccoli, tomato, potato, red & yellow peppers, parsley, cilantro, and citrus (lime, orange, lemon, orange and grapefruit).

DID YOU KNOW?

GROW YOUR OWN BEAN SPROUTS

Sprouts are a great snack. They are yummy in a sandwich instead of lettuce, or just eaten with your fingers! They are full of vitamins and minerals. Best of all? YOU grew them yourself!

Choose small seeds. They sprout faster and are healthier. Plus, larger beans can get moldy. Alfalfa, broccoli, cabbage, small beans, peas, and lentils taste delicious and are easy to grow.

WHAT YOU NEED:

- A clean glass jar
- 1-2 tablespoons of beans or seeds from the market or plant store.
- A small, thin piece of fabric. Gauze that is used for first aid works great.
- A large rubber band or hair tie.

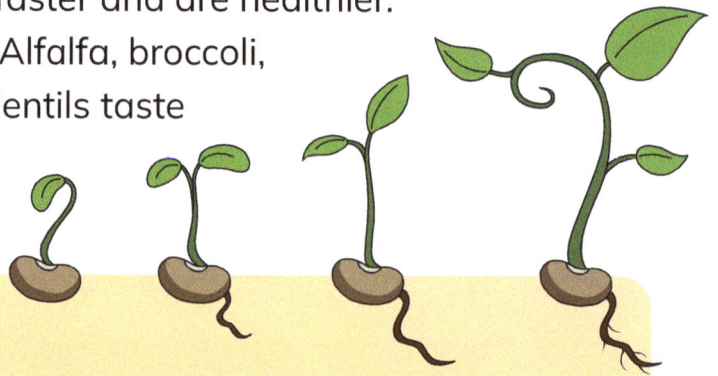

Fill a jar with water. Place fabric over the top. Fix in place with a large rubber band. This lets a little air come in and prevents mold. Soak overnight. Keep the jar away from the sun.

The next day, drain the water through the cloth. Fill with new clean water. Swish the beans around. Drain out all the water.

Rinse and drain two times each day as they start to sprout. This keeps them clean and moist. Even bean sprouts need to drink clean water!

Once they are one to three inches long, rinse, drain and spread them out on a clean paper towel. In about eight hours, they are ready to eat. Store in the refrigerator.

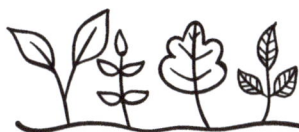

A SEEDLING IS BORN

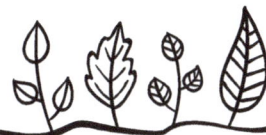

The Life Cycle of a Plant

In less than one week, you can grow your own food! Each day, record what you see. Under each drawing explain what is happening with the seeds.

FLOWER POWER

Next door is a tall hospital. We want to plant a flower bed that will be interesting for the patients when they look down from their windows from up high.

With a ruler, connect the segments* below to create a grid for a pattern.

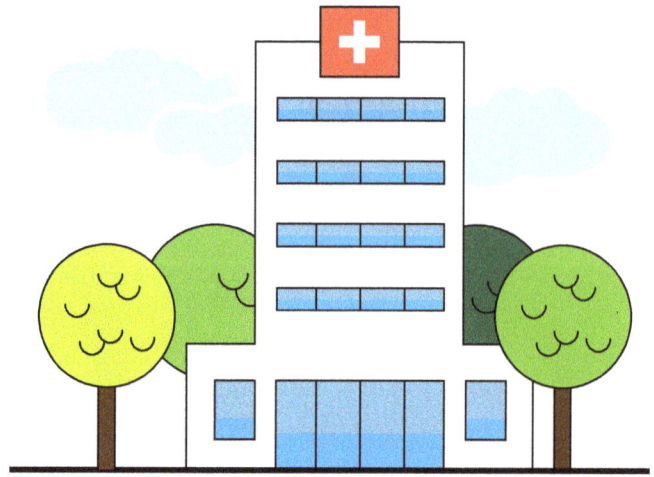

A-I

A-Q

I-Q

E-M

M-U

E-U

A-M

G-S

I-U

E-Q

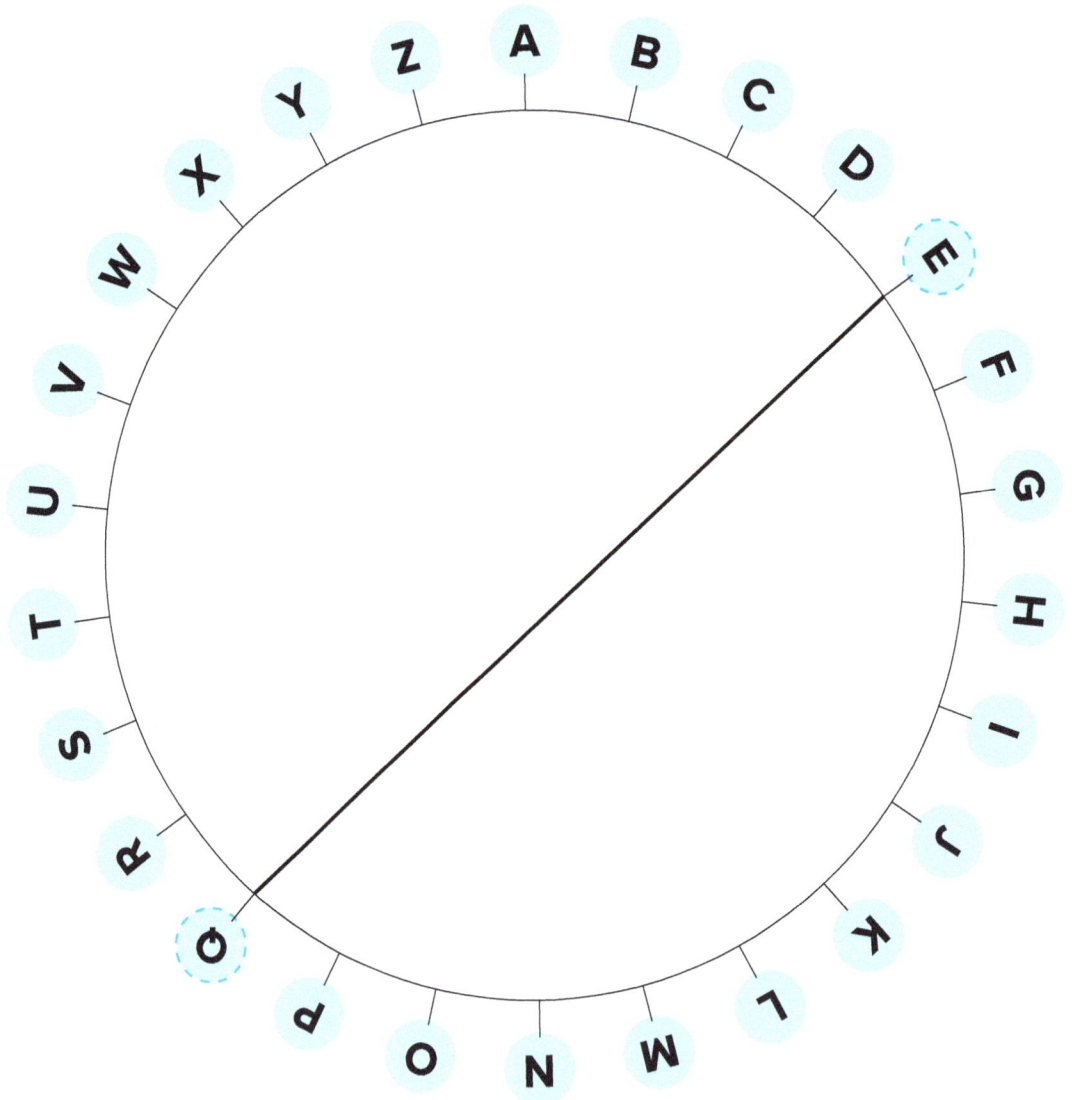

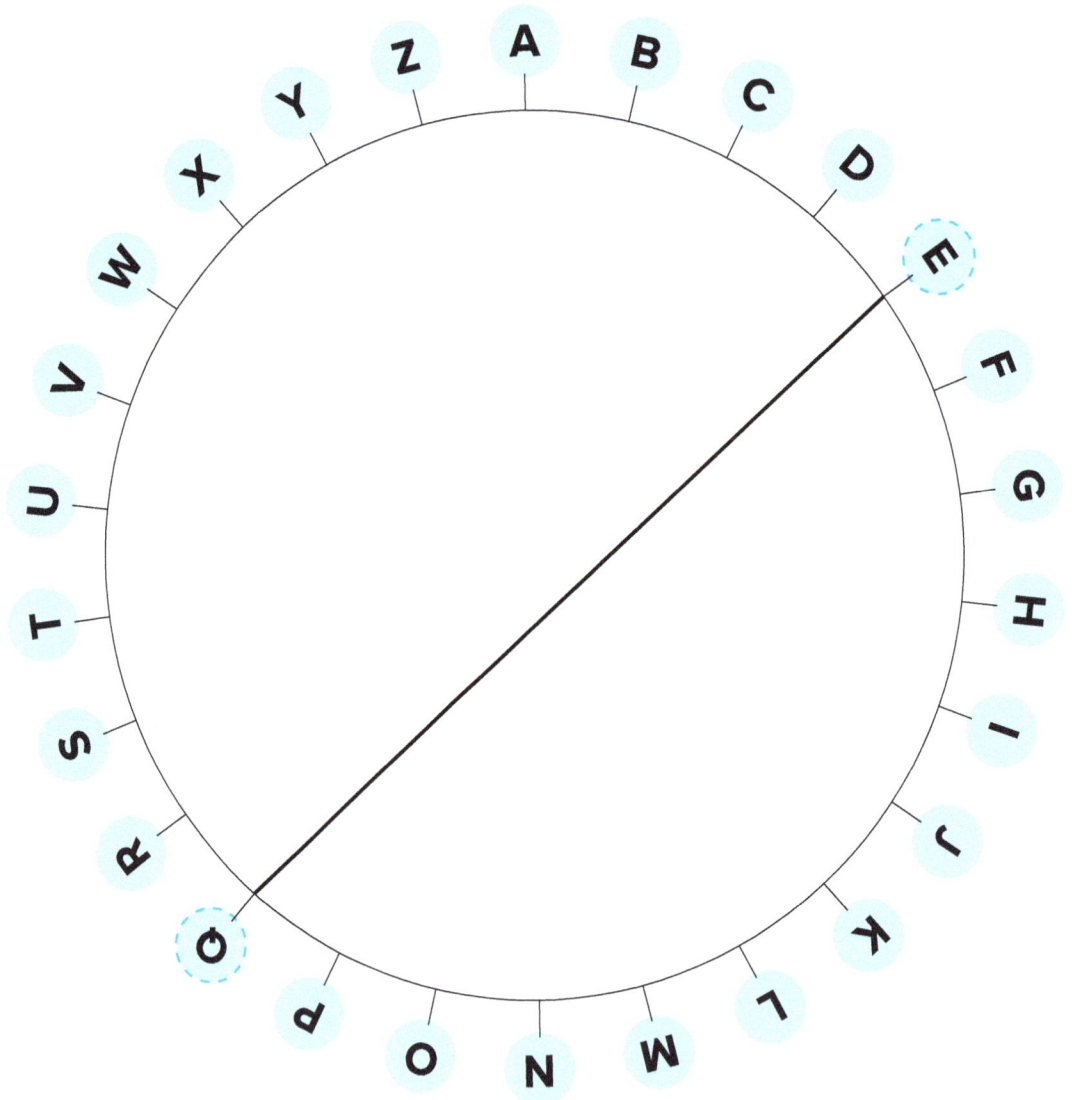

CHECK
IT OUT!

53   *(seg-ment) The line between two end points: E-Q = E———Q

Create patterns using the five different colored flowers we are planting.

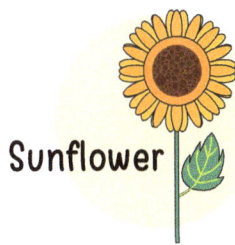

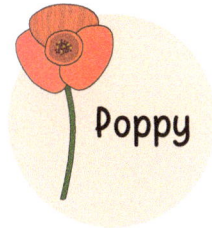

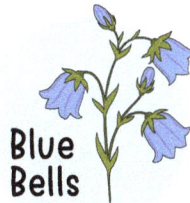

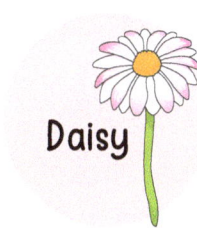

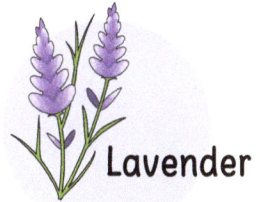

Sunflower

Poppy

Blue Bells

Daisy

Lavender

Make a pattern in the center hexagon with two of the colors.

Use two others for the right angle triangles outside the hexagon.

Use the last color for the obtuse triangles on the outer border.

How many can you find? Remember, different smaller shapes can create bigger shapes. The more you look, the more you will find!

TRIANGLES

Equilateral?
3 equal angles
3 equal sides

Obtuse?
1 angle greater than
90 degrees

Isosceles?
2 equal angles
2 equal sides

Acute?
All angles less than
90 degrees

QUADRILATERALS

Square?
All right angles
All equal sides

Rectangle?
All right angles
2 sets of equal sides
(including squares)

Parallelogram?
4-sided rectangular shape
Opposite sides are parallel
(2 lines with the same distance between them)

Quadrilateral?
4-sided shape

Trapezoid?
Quadrilateral with only one pair
of parallel sides.

Rhombuse?
4-sided shape with opposite equal acute angles
Opposite equal obtuse angles
4 equal sides (including squares)

CHECK IT OUT!

WE GROW LOVE

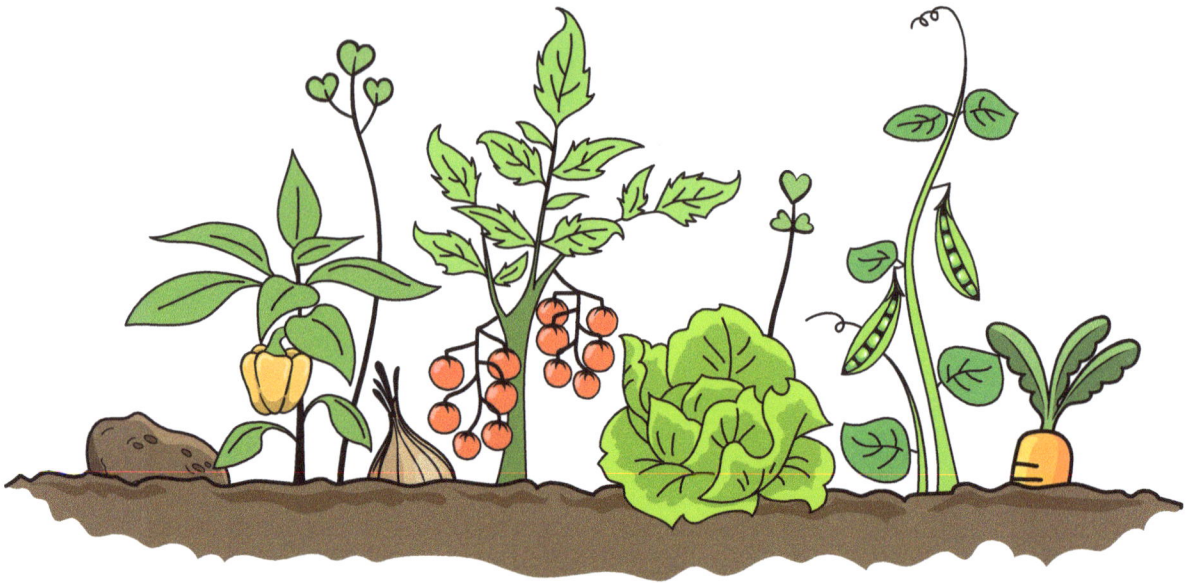

I am always discovering wonderful new flavor combinations. I like to say we grow LOVE in our garden.

I **LOVE** the taste of fresh homegrown delicious summer tomatoes. Add some healthy oil, spices and you have the easiest salad of all to make.

I **LOVE** working in our garden. I love the friends I make and the things I learn.

I **LOVE** watching the plants grow and change everyday.

I **LOVE** finding the first baby strawberries hiding under their big green leaves.

I **LOVE** pulling the best baby carrots and turnips, IN THE WORLD out of the ground.

I **LOVE** that we all worked hard as a team to get started. Now, it is just plain fun.

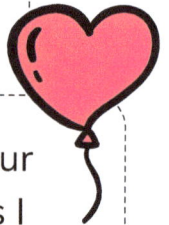

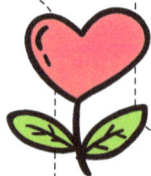

I **LOVE** touching the herbs. The air fills with their smell.

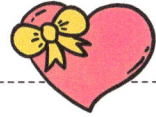

I **LOVE** all the birds and butterflies that now visit our neighborhood.

I **LOVE** growing magic beans. It is seems like magic that from one little bean we can grow buckets of super healthy food! Beans need very little room, since they grow tall instead of wide.

I **LOVE** discovering and eating vegetables that I had never heard of before.

I **LOVE** being proud of what we accomplish.

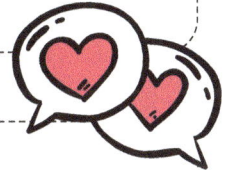

I **LOVE** that our garden overflows with GRRR8 food. We share everything we grow. Some we sell to other people in the community. This helps pay for new seeds and plants.

I **LOVE** that our community garden helps others. We always share our GRRR8 crops with our local food bank.

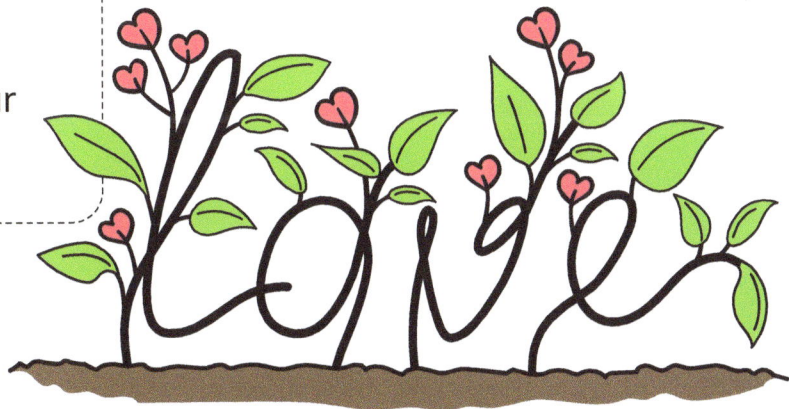

What do I love most?

I **LOVE** working hard, knowing I am helping my family, my classmates and my community eat healthier and live better while having a whole lot of fun!

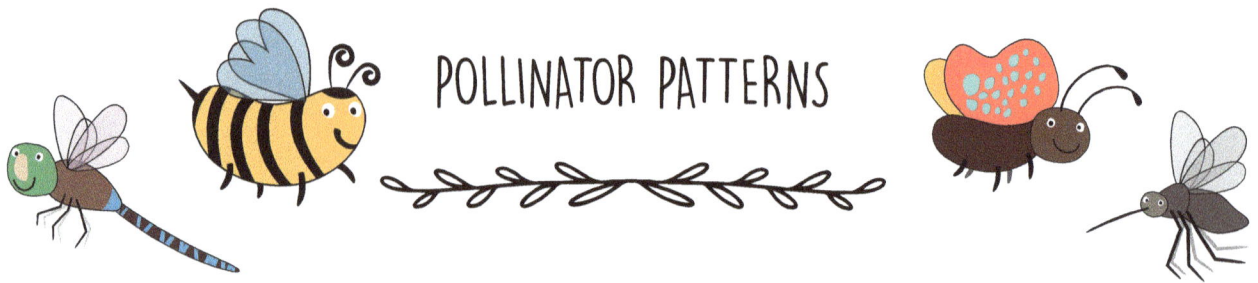

POLLINATOR PATTERNS

I love all the animals that help our garden grow. Worms and snakes make tunnels in the soil, as they eat plant debris*. The tunnels keep the soil soft, letting roots go deeper to find extra water and nutrients. Plus, what goes in, must come out. Worms are mini composters. Plants love their nutrient-rich poop.

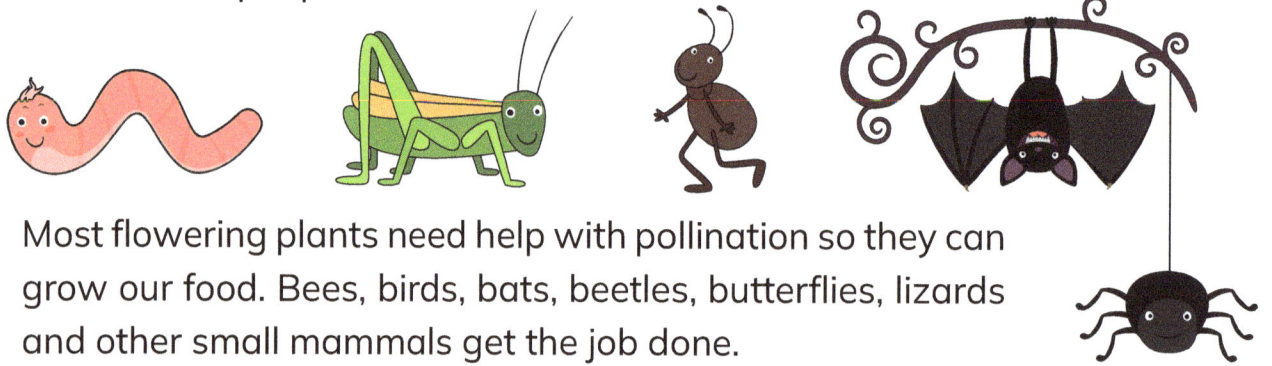

Most flowering plants need help with pollination so they can grow our food. Bees, birds, bats, beetles, butterflies, lizards and other small mammals get the job done.

Wandering from flower to flower, pollen grains stick to their bodies and travel with them to the next flowers. Sadly, this nearly invisible ecosystem is at risk as the earth changes.

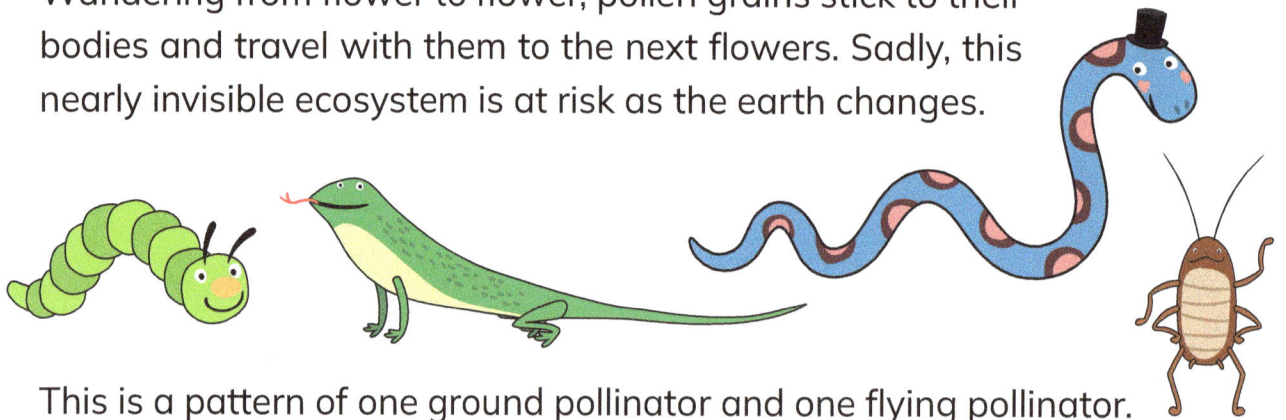

This is a pattern of one ground pollinator and one flying pollinator.

Create a pattern using one ground pollinator and one high flying pollinator.

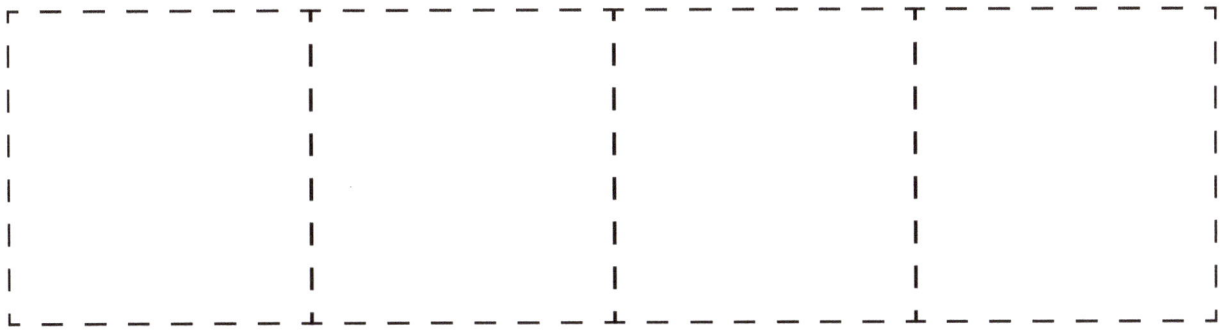

Create a pattern with two bugs.

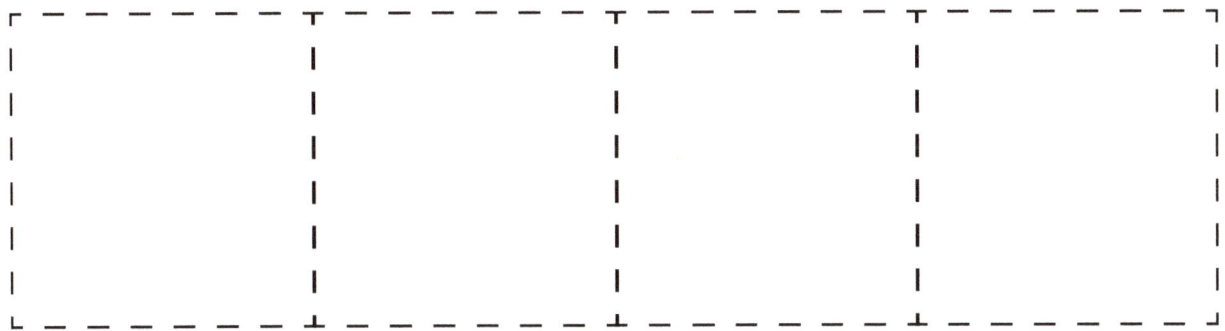

Create a pattern with any two pollinators.

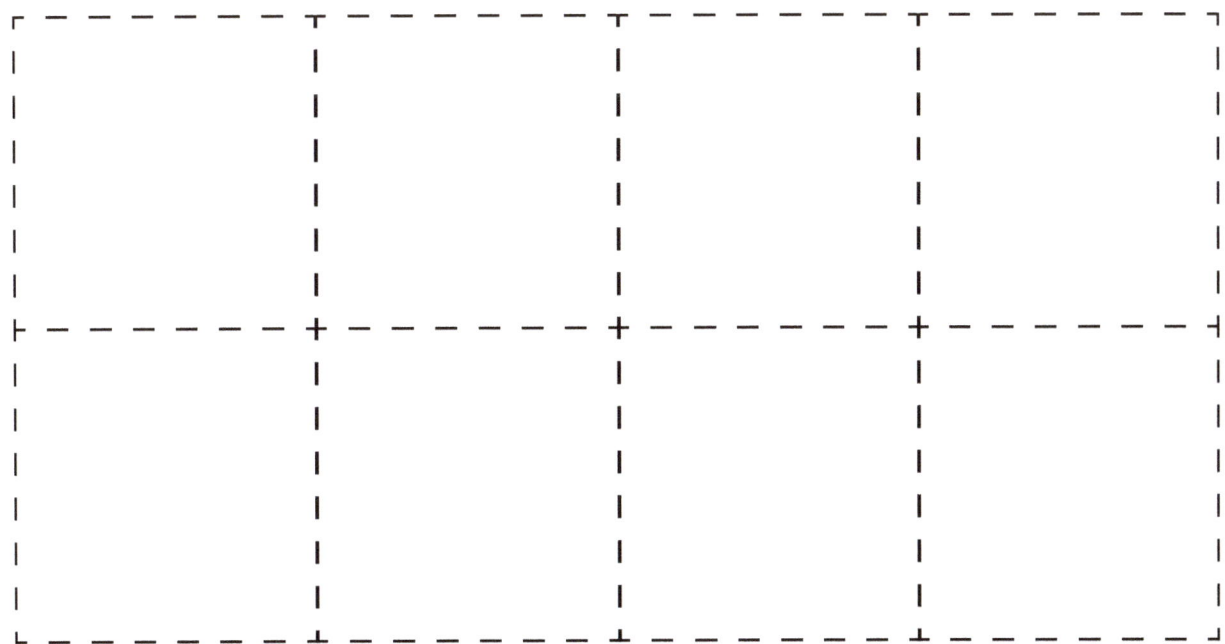

CHECK IT OUT!

HOW DO PLANTS EAT AND DRINK?

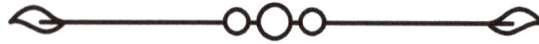

WHAT YOU NEED:

- 1 celery stalk with leaves attached
- Two glasses or jars
- 10 drops of two different food colors
- Water
- A small knife
- Tape
- Crayons or watercolors

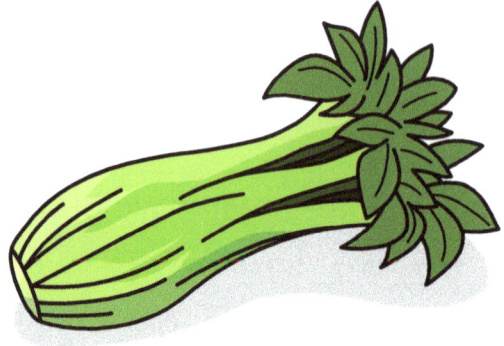

DAY 1   Time: ....   Date: ....

1. Place a piece of tape, horizontally, on the outside of each jar.
2. Mark the tape at 1 inch and 2 inches from the bottom.
3. Cut a slit in of the celery the same height as the glass or jar.
4. Add 2 inches of water. Add food coloring to the water in each jar. Stir to mix.
5. Cut one inch off the bottom of the stalk.
6. Stand one side of the stalk in each jar of water.

HYPOTHESIS

What do you think will happen in the next 24 hours?

....

....

....

CELERY SCIENTIFIC DISCOVERY

Time: _____ **Date:** _____

What changes do you observe?

Is there a change in the water level?

YES   NO

Is there a change in the leaves?

YES   NO

Is there a change in the stem?

YES   NO

What do you see? Draw a picture.

OBSERVATION

Take the stalk out of the jars and cut a inch off the bottom. What do you see in the pieces you cut from the bottom? Draw your discoveries.

CONCLUSION

What do you think happened? Why?

....

....

....

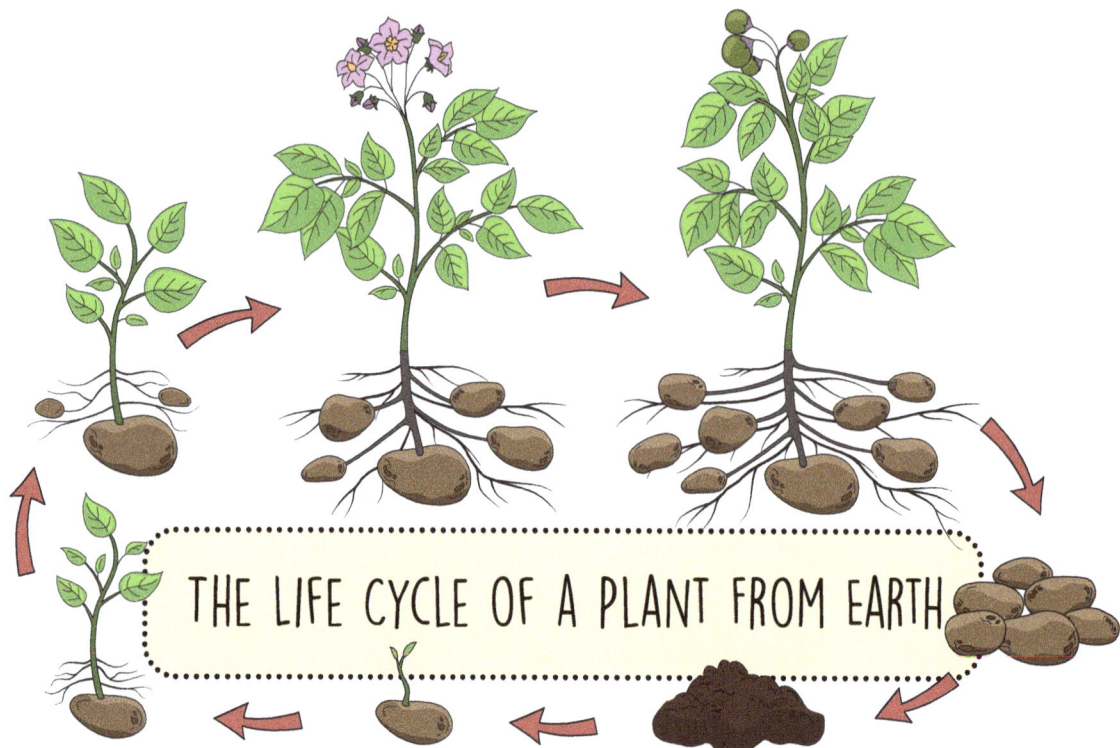

THE LIFE CYCLE OF A PLANT FROM EARTH

There would be no life on the planet without photosynthesis*.

Photosynthesis happens when plants turn sunlight, water (H_2O) and carbon dioxide (CO_2) into their food and ours! Leaves turn bad air (CO_2) into oxygen (O_2) which we need to breathe. Roots soak up nutrients and water from the soil. They travel through the plant through xylem* and phloem* tissues, just like our blood moves through our veins.

Plants become food for us and herbivores*. Herbivores then get eaten by carnivores. In the winter, when the plant dies, it decomposes* into compost.

Compost feeds the soil. Each spring, the cycle starts all over again.

What do you think happens when something super good for us - like a potato - gets covered with mountains of fats from mayo, butter, sour cream, cheese and bacon bits or cooked in oil like chips or fries?   **THINK ABOUT IT!**

*(fow-tow-**SIN**-thah-sis) Plants use the sun to make food from CO_2 and water.
*(**Z.EYE**-lum) Moves water and nutrients up from the roots through the plant.
*(**FLOW**-em) Helps spread the nutrients from the leaves. *(dee-come-**POZE**) to become rotten or decay.
*(**UR**-bah-vor) A creature that only eats plants. *(**CAR**-na-vor) A creature that mostly eats meat or fish.

THE POTATO PLANT

Fill in the blanks with the words below. Color in the drawing.

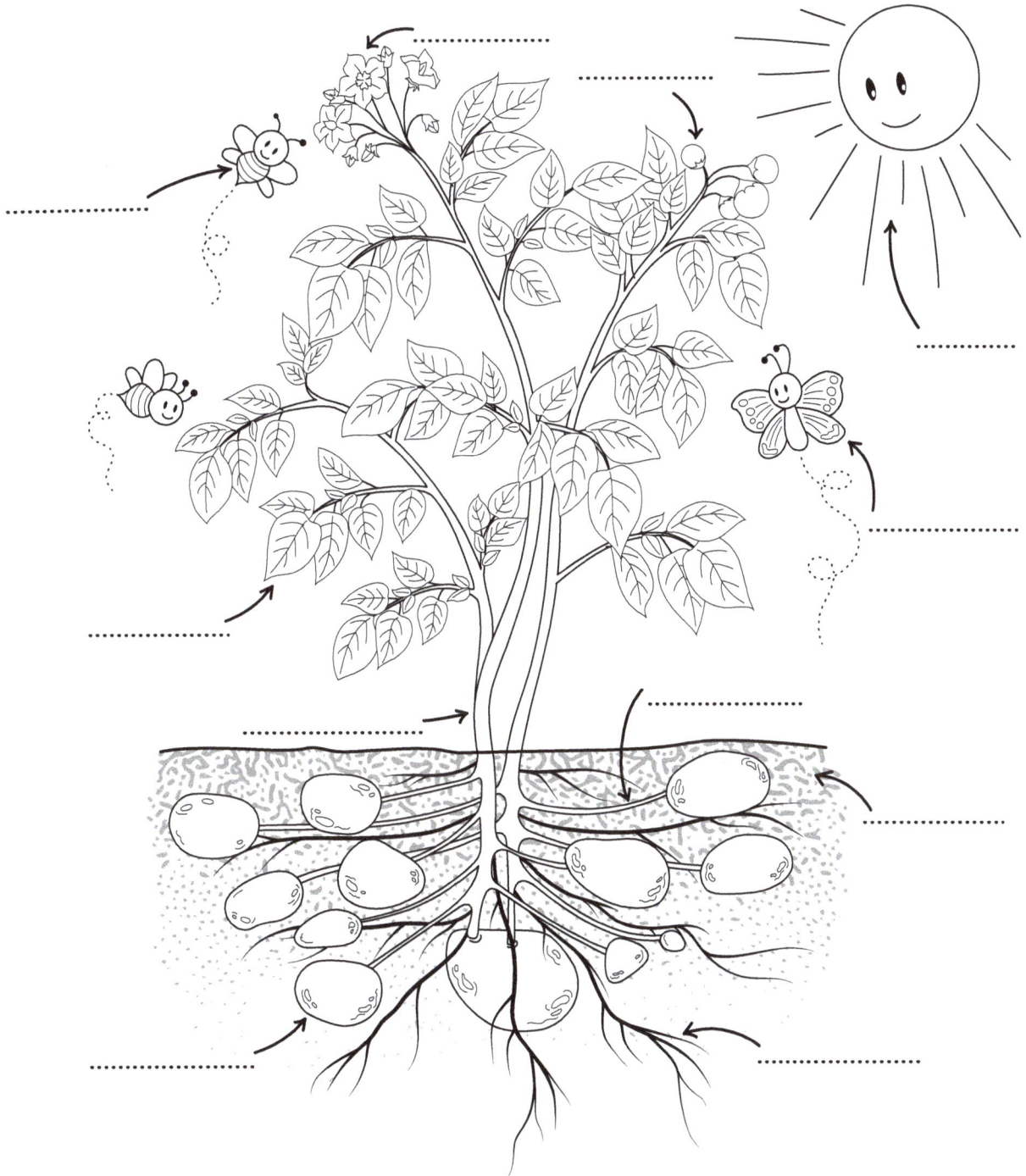

photosynthesis - compost - nutrients - stem- root water - leaf -
butterfly - tuber - sun - air - flower - earth - bee   **WORD BANK**

CHECK
IT OUT!

GROW A POTATO VINE

WHAT YOU NEED:

- One potato
- 4 toothpicks
- Wide-mouthed clear jar or drinking glass

READY, SET, GO!

1. Poke toothpicks into the potato on 4 sides near the top.
2. Place the potato in the jar and fill with water. Toothpicks should sit on the top of the jar, keeping part of the potato above the water.
3. Place the jar on a window ledge. Change the water each day. Roots will start to form after a few days.

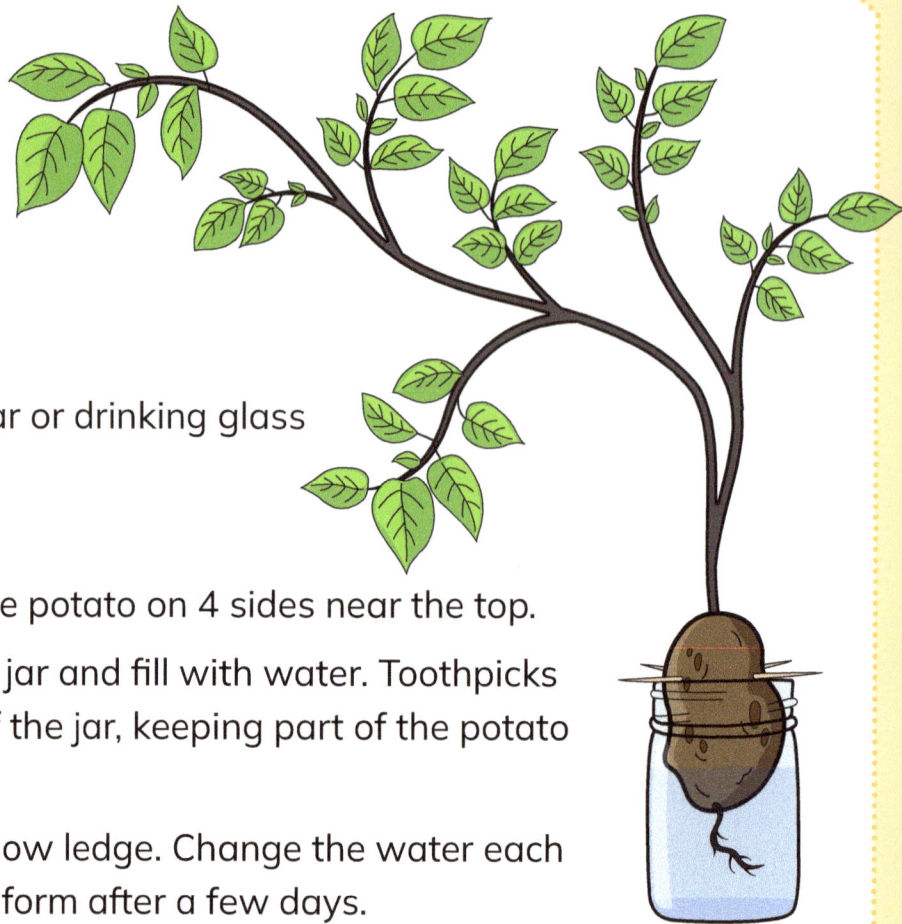

Keep a log as the potato changes.
Write down your discoveries or make drawings below.

HAVE FUN!

WEEK ONE	WEEK TWO	WEEK THREE

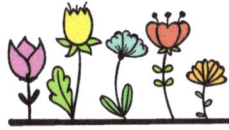

HELP MY GARDEN GROW!

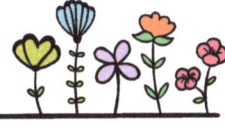

Discover what we need for a great garden.

P M O S C O T __ __ __ __ __ __ __

Rotted plant parts (leaves, grass, fruits and veggies) added to improve garden soil.

L L E I T S R __ __ __ __ __ __ __

Support for climbing plants made from narrow pieces of metal, wood or plastic.

L I S O __ __ __ __

Top layer of earth where plants grow.

L V E G A R __ __ __ __ __ __

Tiny rocks used to make dry paths and drain soil.

C G R A O N I __ __ __ __ __ __ __

Plants and animals raised without the use of chemicals.

N G M A E I E R T __ __ __ __ __ __ __ __ __

When a seed starts to sprout tiny roots and leaves.

N T I U E N T R S __ __ __ __ __ __ __ __

Vitamins and minerals (absorbed through roots or blood) used to grow strong.

P P A E L __ __ __ __ __

A round, red fruit that is great for your health and your teeth.

compost - enrich - drainage - germinate - gravel -
apple - soil - trellis - organic - nutrients

WORD BANK

64

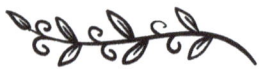 ACROSS →

1. The natural process of breaking down dead plants or animals.

2. Plants that have remained the same for over 50 years.

3. Fresh vegetables or fruit.

4. A long-handled tool used for digging by being pushed into the ground with the foot.

5. The science and art of growing plants.

6. When pollen is transfered from the stamen to the pistel on a flower.

7. A plant that lives for one year.

8. A plant that does not need another plant's pollen to make fruit.

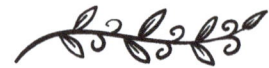 DOWN ↓

1. Plants that are used to give flavor to food or used as medicine.

2. Something safe to eat.

3. A plant that lives more than two years.

4. A long-handle tool used for digging, lifting, and scooping.

5. Tiny young plants grown from seeds.

6. Genetically Modified Organism (G.M.O.). Something living that has been changed through science.

7. Result of water and soil mixing, especially after rain.

Mud - Produce - G.M.O. - Horticulture (**HORE**-ti-cull-chur) - Pollination Herbs (errbs) - Shovel - Seedlings - Heirloom (hair-loom) - Edible Self-pollination - Decompose (dee-come-**POZE**) - Perennial (pah-**RIN**-ee-al) - Spade - Annual (an-**NEW**-al)

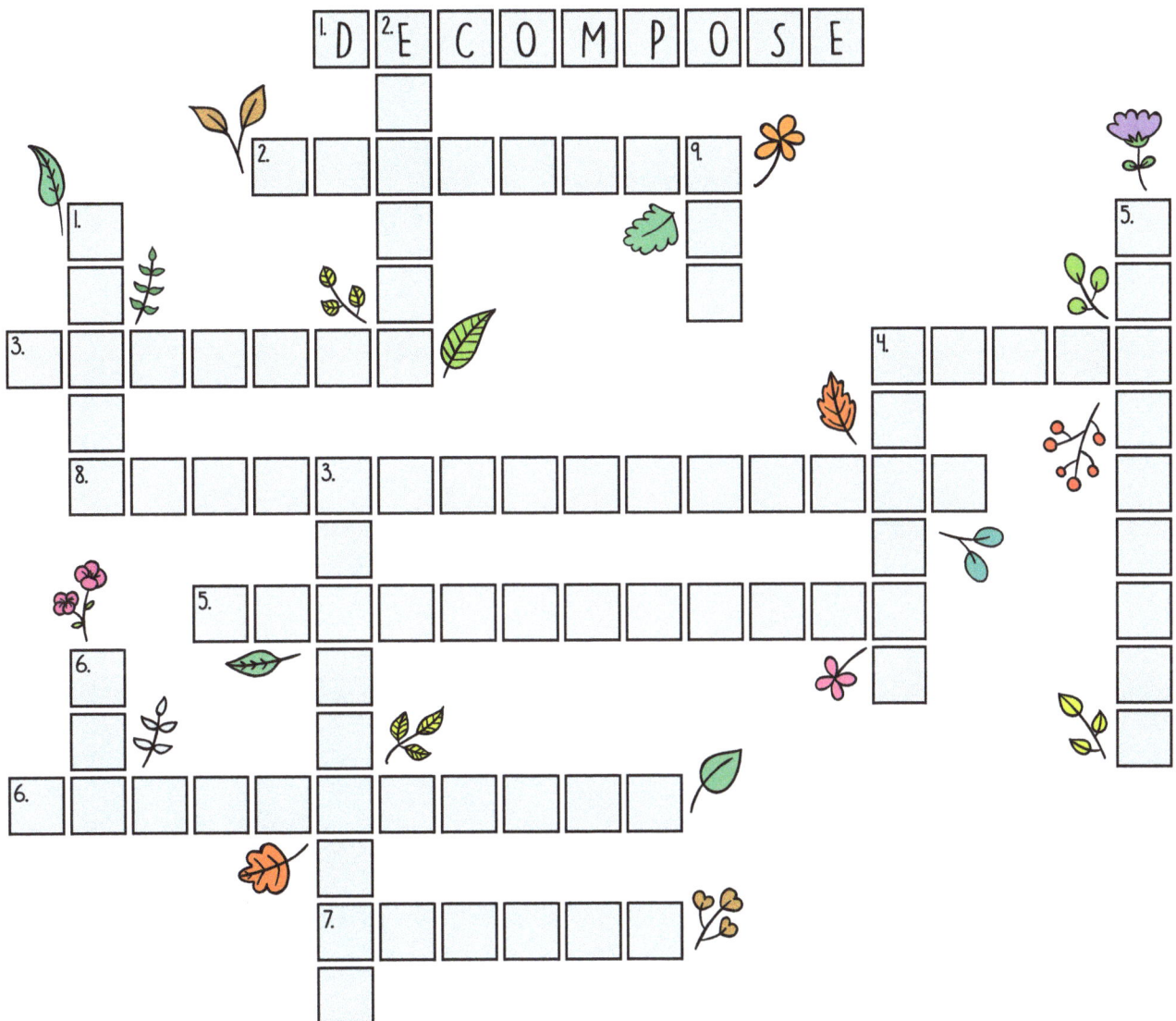

1. D 2.E C O M P O S E

DINNER LIKE A DUCK

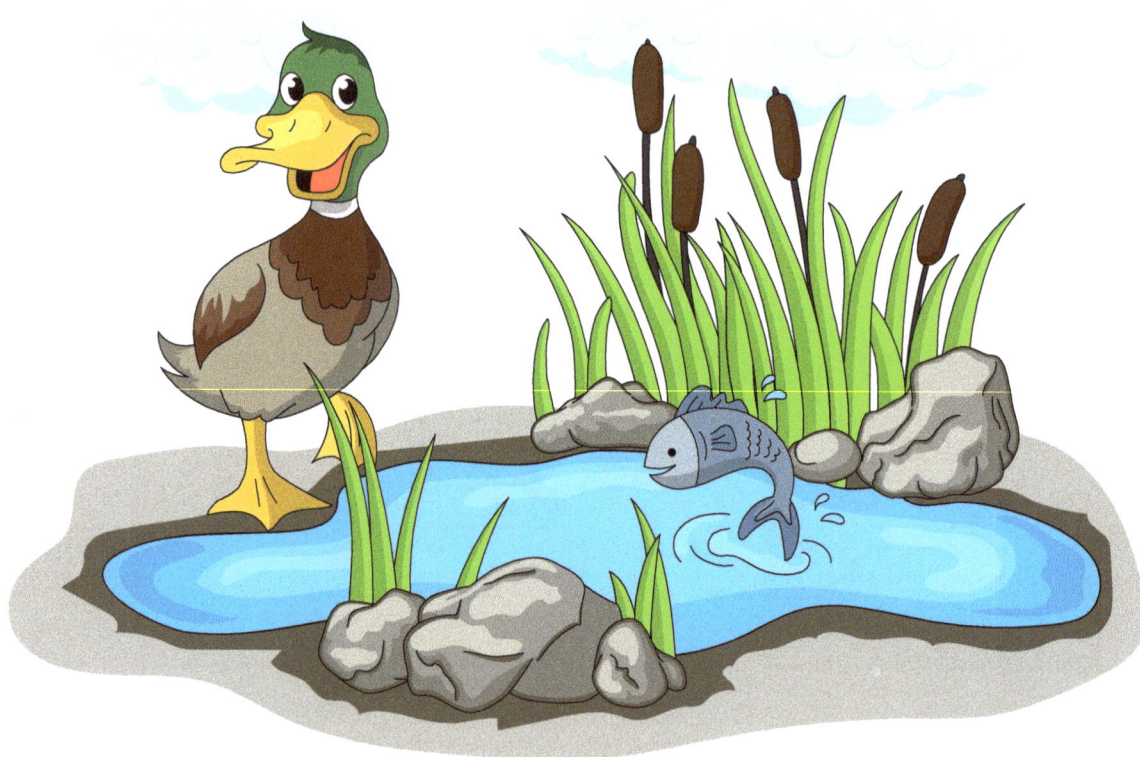

We walk into the kitchen and hand Mom our garden basket filled with GRRR8 things from our garden.

"My goodness, what are we having for dinner tonight?" Mom asks as she trades us each a glass of water for our basket.

She looks at our treasures. *"What about a version of Sky and Earth? Spinach, mashed potatoes and a delicious, bright orange and green salad with carrots, peas and mint. Baked apples with honey-yogurt topping makes a yummy dessert. If we add hard-boiled eggs, we have a perfect dinner,"* Mom suggests.

Everything sounds GRRR8!

"Do you know why dinosaurs eat raw meat?"

"Because they never learned to cook!"

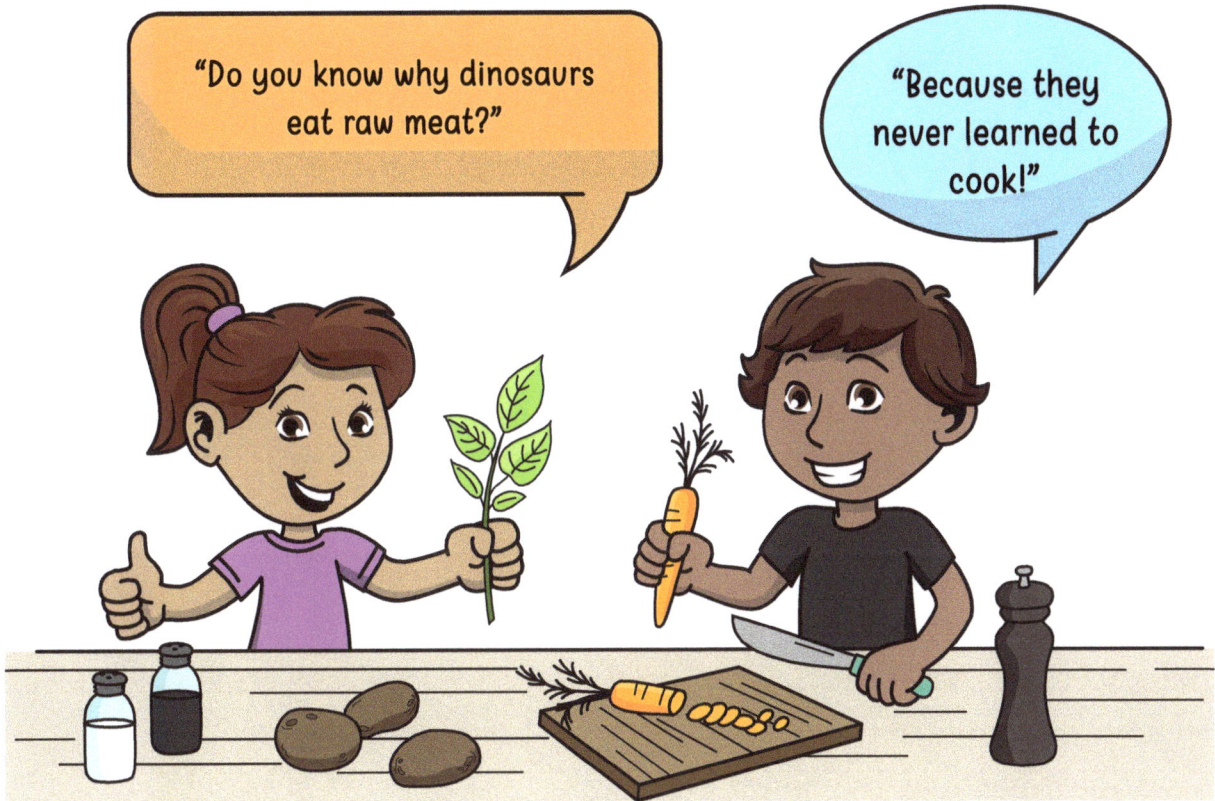

As we chop, peel, grate, smash, and mix, we tell Mom about all the great things we discovered and learned at the garden. We tell her about working with our friends and all the GRRR8 food ready for harvesting. We talk about the seeds we planted and the young plants growing in the beds.

It was a fun day.

What do dinosaurs do when they sleep? They DIE-NO-snore!

Cost per person for Heaven and Earth:

Spinach:	10 cents
Potato:	15 cents,
Egg:	20 cents
Carrot:	10 cents
Apple:	40 cents
Yogurt topping:	15 cents

Approximate Total: $1.10

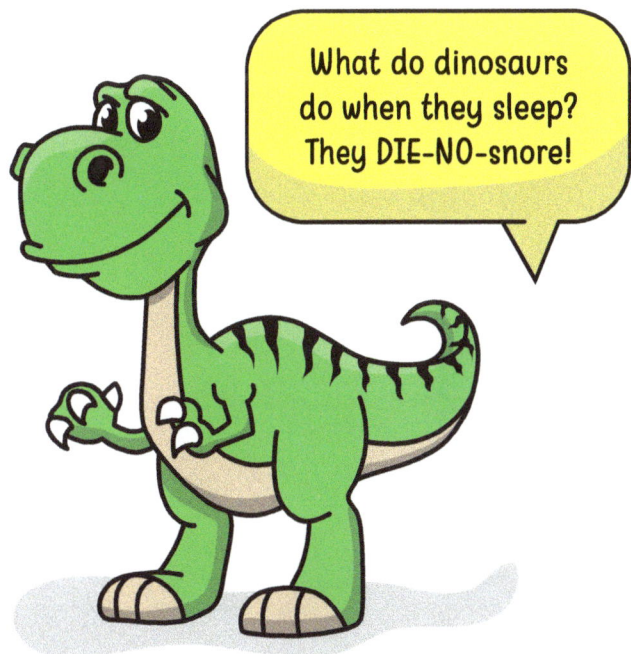

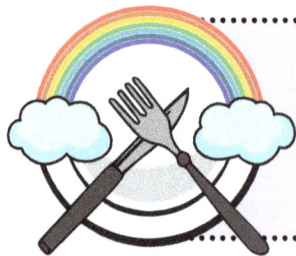

EVERY BITE MATTERS!
EAT RAINBOWS

PROTEIN Plant-based sources like beans, oats, quinoa, soy, nuts, seeds, lentils, broccoli and green beans are super GRRR8 power boosters.

Fish, chicken, turkey and eggs are yummy in salads or straight on your plate. Fatty meats like hamburger are OK sometimes but a grilled chicken burger is Happy Heart smarter.

Processed meats like hot dogs, bologna, bacon and sausage can cause big heath problems.

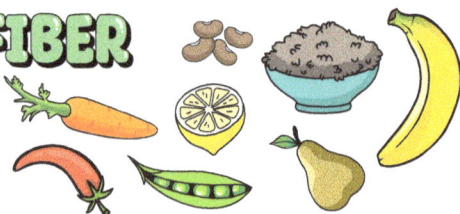

FIBER Fruits, vegetables and grains are GRRR8 nutrition and fiber. Your blood says "thank you" when you choose brown rice, whole grain breads and pastas.

FAT Good Healthy Heart oil from plants or fish each day helps our body absorb minerals, nutrients and vitamins.

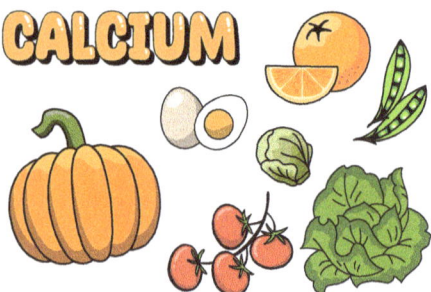

CALCIUM Extremely important for strong bone growth - dairy and plant 'milks', sugar-free yogurt, cheese, beans, lentils, pumpkin, tofu, greens, eggs, sardines, canned salmon (because you eat their tiny bones) are all GRRR8 choices.

VEGETABLES

Eat as many vegetables as you like but watch what you put on top. Check out: **Happy Healthy Heart Super Me** Ranch dressing on page 89.

FRUIT

Fruit is important, but in smaller amounts than veggies because fruit, especially grapes, has a lot of natural sugar. Too much of any kind of sugar makes it hard for your body to stay balanced.

GRAINS

Choose whole grain breads, pasta, or tortillas. Once you get use to the nutty rich taste, you will love it. One slice of bread is all kids need per meal.

JUST SOMETIMES

Salt, sugar, sweets, cakes, candy, chips, processed and fried foods: it is best to keep this group the smallest.

HERBS & SPICES

These add lots of GRRR8 flavor and help keep us healthy. Since early days, herbs and spices have been used for everything from keeping away bugs, killing germs and medicine. Adding spices instead of salt or sugar is a win-win.

REMEMBER
Always check the ingredients for hidden salt & sugars!

CHECK IT OUT!

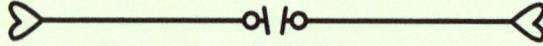

EATING SMART

Just like a seesaw - It's one big balancing act

A WELL BALANCED MEAL

"Eating Smart" means eating a balanced meal made up of different Healthy Happy Heart foods. Use our kid portion map at the front of the book for portion sizes.

Half   Quarter

Let your plate and fractions be your guide: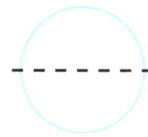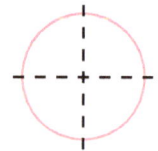

The best plate fraction balance is 1/2 vegetables/fruit (eat more vegetables than fruit), 1/4 whole grains, 1/4 protein, one serving of calcium and a little healthy plant oil.

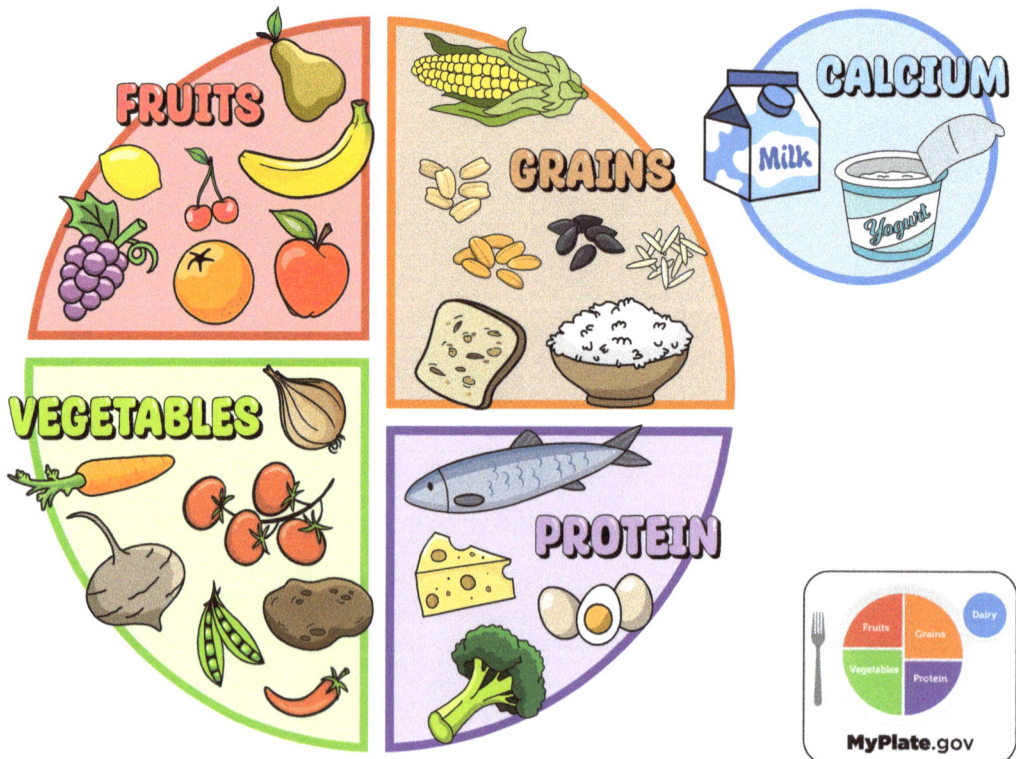

CHECK IT OUT!

BE MY GUEST

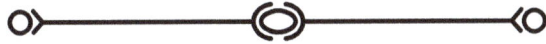

America needs healthy kids to grow up and take care of our country. If a famous athlete was invited to your school for lunch, what special meal would you serve?

Remember, athletes - like us - need to be healthy and strong to do their job. Make sure to serve something delicious and nutritious.

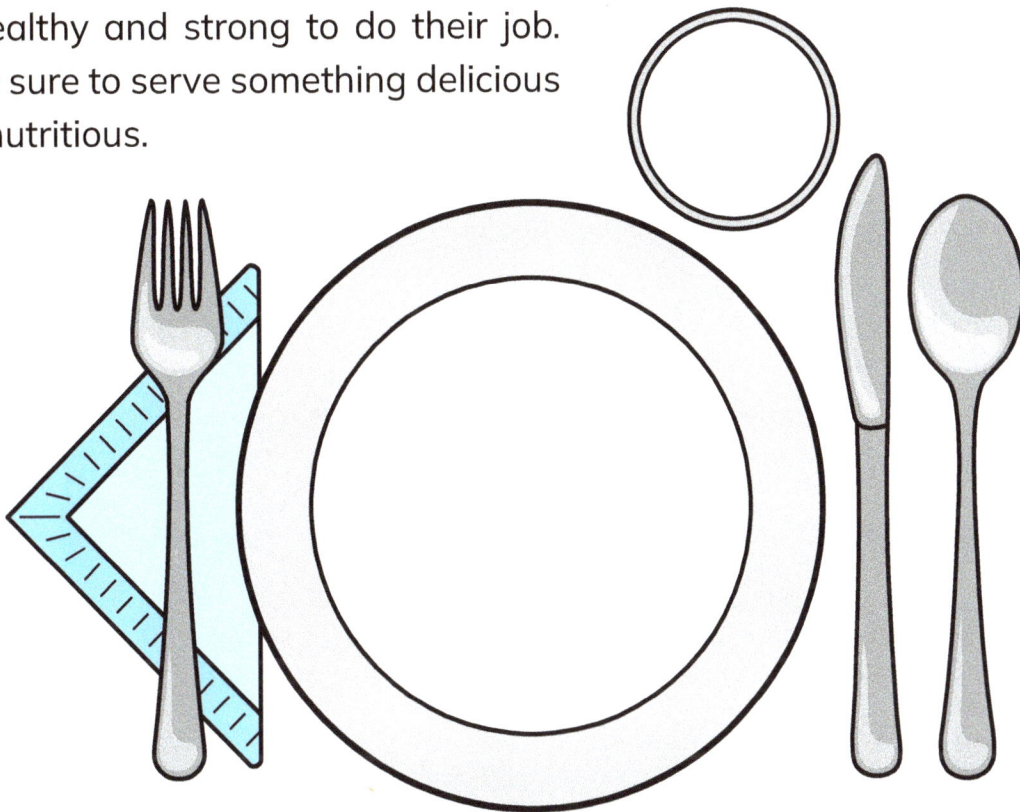

		How would you prepare each dish? Fresh, steamed, roasted? Would you add other ingredients?
Drink		
Healthy Protein		
Vegetable		
Whole Grain		
Fruit		

VENN DIAGRAM

Compare Basic Plant and Human Needs

How many things can you think of that are necessary for plants and humans to have a healthy life cycle? Fill in the diagram. In the middle, draw or write the needs humans and plants have in common.

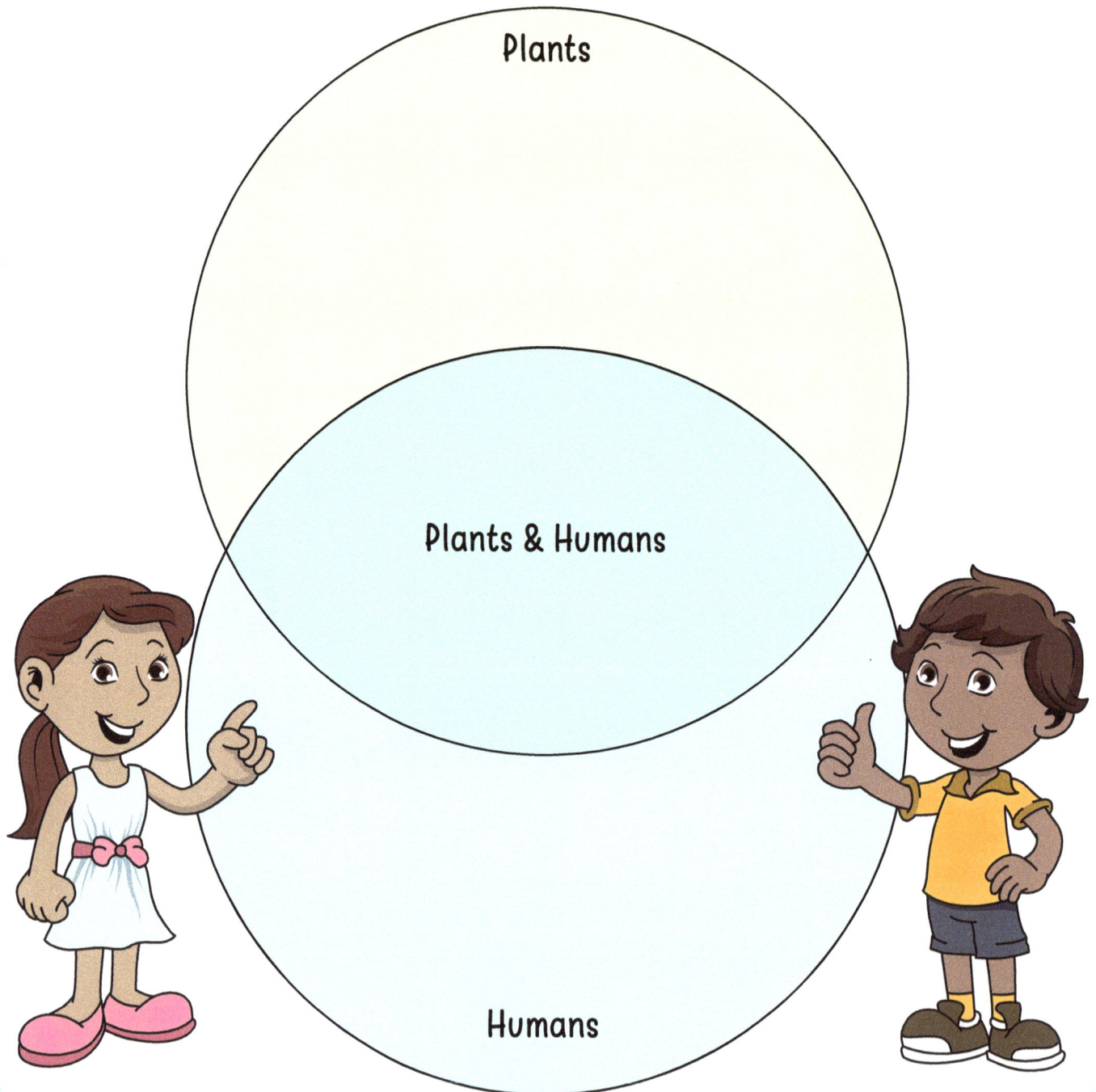

Plants

Plants & Humans

Humans

HEALTHY HAPPY HEART SHOPPING BUDGET

Knowing how to stretch your money is a very important life skill.

Imagine doing the shopping your own shopping. You have $2.00.
Make the smartest **Happy Healthy Heart** choices to make you GRRR8.*

Things to think about:

- Does this item give me **GRRR8 Happy Healthy Heart** points?
- Is it worth my money? Which is cheaper? Fresh, frozen or canned?
- Store brands usually cost less than the national famous brands.
- Prepared foods, pre-cut and cleaned fruits and veggies, and snack foods like chips, cookies, sodas, etc. are all very expensive food points.

1 serving of pre-washed carrots costs _____.
1 serving of whole carrots costs _____.

....

....

....

....

....

....   **+**   .... **=** ....
TOTAL   TOTAL   GRAND TOTAL

Pineapple: $0.30 Fresh/ $1.57 Fresh pre-cut / $0.83 Frozen/ $0.28 Canned

Corn: $0.18 Canned/ $0.25 Frozen

Carrots: $0.12 Fresh pre-cut / $0.09 Whole fresh / $0.25 Sliced frozen / $0.25 Sliced canned

Spinach: $0.40 Canned / $0.35 Frozen / $1.00 Fresh

Peas: $0.25 Frozen

Yellow potato: $0.30

Sweet potato: $0.50

Store brand bottle of soda: $0.10

National brand of soda: $0.20

100% Apple juice: $0.20

Egg: $0.20

Cottage cheese: $0.25

Greek yogurt: $0.72

Potato chips(13): $0.25

Roasted peanuts: $0.14

Whole oats: $0.13

Canned beans: $0.22

Corn tortilla: $0.06

Muffin: $1.25

Donut: $1.00

Boneless-skinless chicken breast: $1.00 Fresh / $0.83 Frozen

Boneless-skinless thigh: $0.88 Fresh / $0.77 Frozen

Chicken legs: $0.20

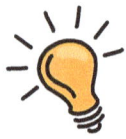

SO MANY NEW WORDS AND IDEAS!

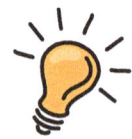

You have learned so much already.
See how many of the words you can find below.

H	A	P	P	Y	R	H	E	A	T	H	Y	A	H	B
A	V	E	O	E	T	A	B	L	E	X	O	I	L	S
N	S	A	T	I	A	T	E	N	E	R	G	Y	U	M
T	W	S	A	L	A	D	G	H	R	J	U	M	P	E
I	D	D	T	C	U	C	U	M	B	E	R	R	Y	V
O	W	S	O	U	P	I	G	M	E	N	T	S	D	I
X	C	O	L	O	R	S	I	M	M	U	N	E	A	T
I	R	U	H	K	U	L	S	Y	S	T	E	M	A	A
D	U	P	B	G	M	E	T	A	B	O	L	I	S	M
A	N	U	T	S	H	E	L	P	B	R	A	I	N	I
N	C	E	M	R	T	P	T	P	R	O	T	E	I	N
T	S	B	I	G	G	O	A	L	O	L	O	V	E	S
E	Y	E	L	L	O	W	B	E	F	S	M	A	R	T
N	F	B	K	C	O	W	L	O	M	E	A	T	S	A
T	B	L	O	O	D	C	E	L	L	S	T	I	M	E
F	R	U	I	T	W	A	T	E	R	T	O	X	I	N

toxin - dream - happy - color - brain - love - bumblebee - nut goal - table
- system - rest - protein - smart - water fruit - jump - salad - blood - help
- satiate - yellow - immune - energy - berry - metabolism
- cell - nut...+ so many more!

WORD BANK

What Goes in Must Come Out

A toilet is like an underwater health report card. Understanding what you see or smell, lets you know how well you are taking care of your body.

The color, smell and shape of pee and poop change because of exercise, what we eat and drink or if there is a health issue. Things like red beets, medicines or vitamins can change how they look or smell. It is important to know what is normal for you.

Usually, pee is a light yellow color. A dark yellow says, "Drink more water!"

The intestines work like a garbage disposal, turning leftover food into poop. Poop tells you things, too. Poop should come out pretty easily, comfortably and a couple of inches long. It shouldn't be too hard, soft or slimy.

Weird shapes say, "More water, fiber or exercise, please."
Hot dog or snake shape? A+

Please Tell an Adult if:
- If something hurts coming or smells weird.
- Your pee is dark brown.
- Your poop looks like baby food or a milkshake.

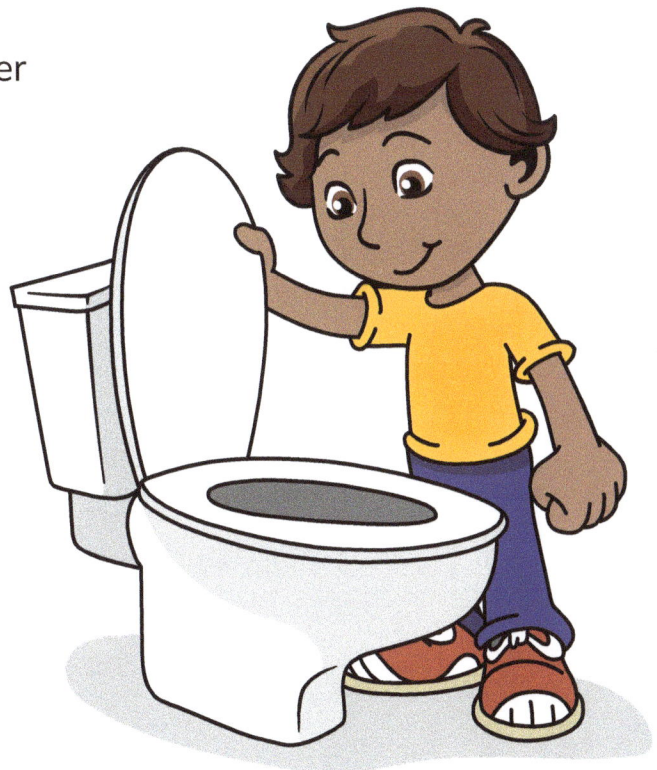

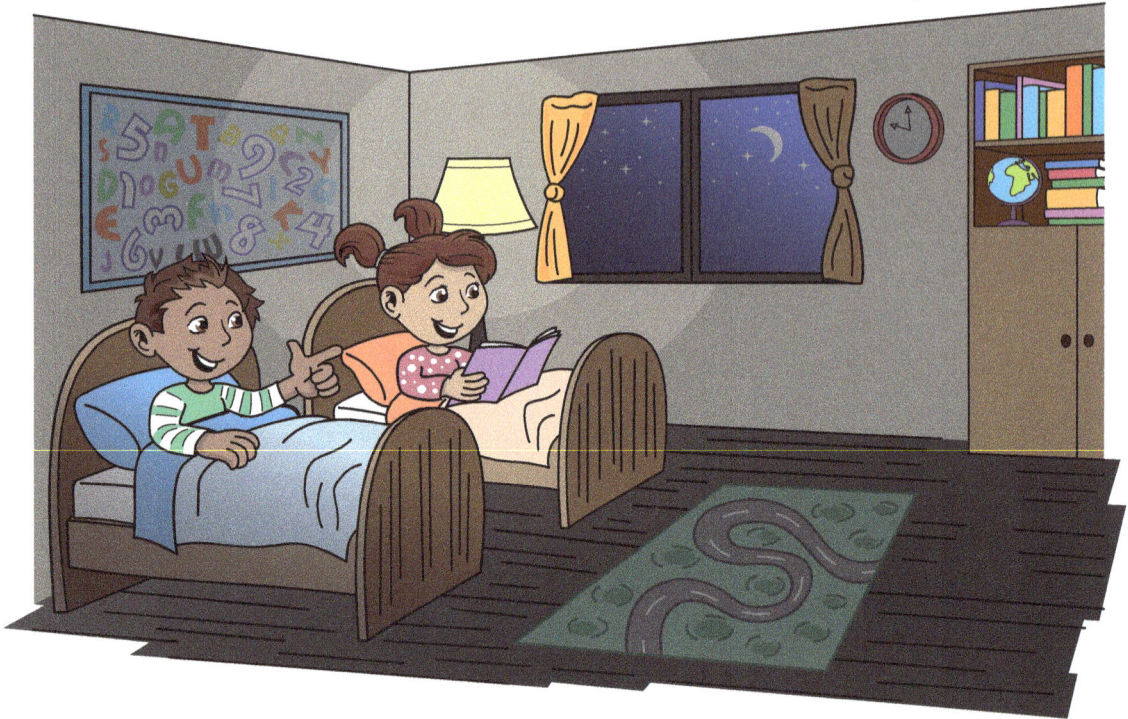

Another great day has come to an end. I learned new things and made GRRR8 memories. *"Good night, best brother ever,"* I call to BB.

"Good night, best little sister!"
he laughs back.

We giggle as I put down my book, turn off my light and wonder what discoveries await me in the morning.

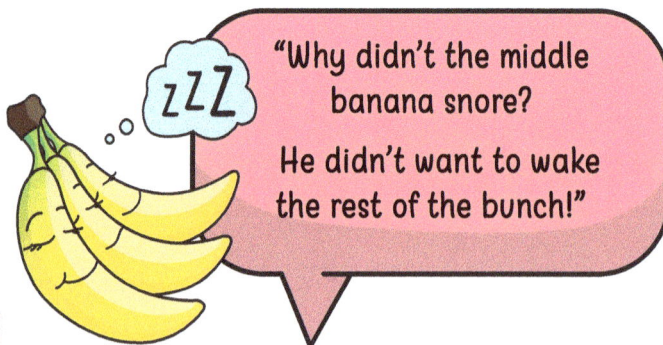

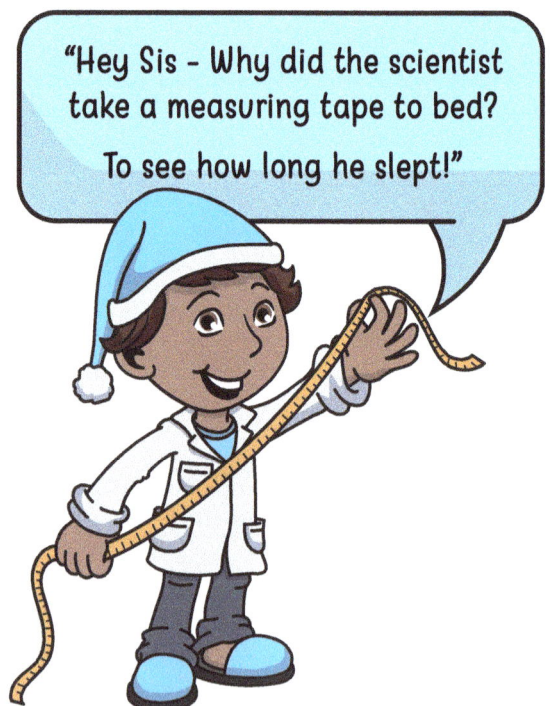

"Hey Sis - Why did the scientist take a measuring tape to bed?

To see how long he slept!"

"Why didn't the middle banana snore?

He didn't want to wake the rest of the bunch!"

CHECK IT OUT!

LOOK HOW MUCH SMARTER I AM NOW!

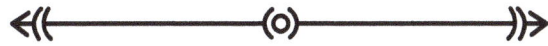

Discover how much you have learned.
Pick the goals you now know are important.
Cross out the not-helping choices.
Explain why you picked your **GRRR8** choices.

Things I can do as I grow to help keep me on my GRRR8 path are:

....
....
....
....
....
....
....
....
....
....

| Help in school. | Love the library. | Dream. | Be the best student I can be. |

| Eat healthy food. | Learn all I can. | Play lots of games. | Eat lots of candy. |

| Drink lots of soda. | Drink lots of water. | Eat 5 fruits and veggies every day. |

| Do all my homework. | Exercise every day. | Stay up late. | Read lots of books. |

| Learn everything I can on interesting subjects. | Get 8 hours of sleep each night. |

| Come to school each day prepared to give my best. | Forget to do my homework. |

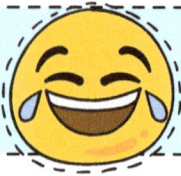

LOOK WHAT I NOW KNOW!

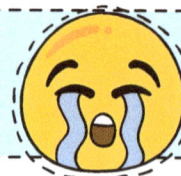

Now, add a smiley 😄 or sad 😔 faces and
two more tricks you have learned.

- ☐ _____
- 😄 Drinking lots of water
- ☐ Eat sweets every day
- ☐ Eat veggies every day
- ☐ Brush my teeth morning and night
- ☐ Play electronics
- ☐ Do 50 jumping jacks a day
- ☐ Stay up late at night
- ☐ Help make fresh food
- ☐ Always salt my food
- ☐ Read books
- ☐ Sing

- ☐ _____
- ☐ Dream
- ☐ Hop
- ☐ Be grumpy
- ☐ Dance
- ☐ Skip school
- ☐ Spend lots of time on a phone
- ☐ Drink soda
- ☐ Learn to cook
- ☐ Play sports
- ☐ Wash my hands when I come home from school, before eating and after using the restroom

I AM HELPING MY BODY BE GRRR8!

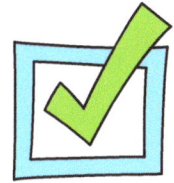

Wow, **SUPER ME-4-LIFE** tricks I learned:

	Mon	Tue	Wed	Thu	Fri	Sat	Sun
I laughed, danced, jumped and smiled today.							
I ate less salt, sugar and fat filled food.							
I drank enough water.							
I slept at least 8 hours.							
I exercised at least 30 minutes.							
I washed my hands after using the bathroom, coming home from school, before cooking and eating.							
I made the best Happy Healthy Heart food choices I could today.							
I ate 5 vegetables and fruit servings!							
I brushed my teeth at least 2 times.							
I learned something new today.							
I listened to my body.							
I was proud of myself.							
I was thankful for something.							
I focused on good thoughts.							
I was kind.							

A JAPANESE HAIKU 4 YOU!

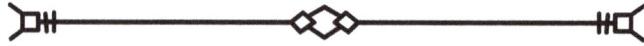

Haiku poems are short and fun to write. They are only three lines long and are based on syllables.

Line one has five syllables. Line two has seven syllables.

The poem ends with five syllables in line three.

Write a Haiku about something you learned.

Up, down, Up, down, Up (5)

Jumping makes me laugh all day (7)

Playing together (5)

Running and jumping (5)

Super Me helps me be strong (7)

Smiling all day long (5)

READY, SET, LET'S COOK

"Knock - knock, who's there?
- Lettuce... - Lettuce who?
- Lettuce in and you will know!"

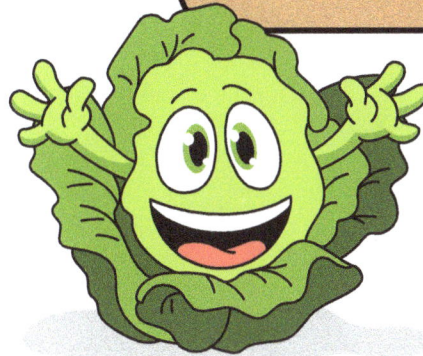

Pantry and fridge items to keep ready:

▶ **Natural vinegar**

▶ **Spices**

▶ **Coconut or date sugar, agave syrup or natural honey**

▶ **Mustard** (Sugar free!)

▶ **Canned goods:** water packed tuna, beans, tomatoes, pumpkin.

▶ **Whole grains:** pasta, bread and tortillas.

▶ **Quinoa** is GRRR8! It looks like rice or pasta but it is a super protein; loaded with vitamins, minerals and fiber.

▶ **Oats:** Rolled oats are GRRR8!

▶ **Nuts:** easy to grab for a quick snack at home or on the run. 1 handful = 1`serving.

▶ **100% Nut butter**

▶ **100% Applesauce:** a sweetener for cooking, baking, in cereal, on cottage cheese, or to eat as-is.

▶ **Eggs:** always ready for a GRRR8 easy meal. Add one to a salad or to grab-on-the-go.

▶ **Fruits/veggies:** 100% fresh, frozen or canned.

▶ **Potatoes, carrots and cabbage:** Cheap and healthy.

▶ **Sugar Free Yogurt:** snack, make creamy snacks, dips or for cooking.

▶ **Milk:** cow, goat, plant based or powdered; for drinking or cooking.

▶ **Cheese:** natural hard and cottage.

▶ **Healthy Happy Heart Made@ Home dips and salsa -** GRRR8 on everything. (p 113)

82

TOOLS OF THE TRADE & QUICK TRICKS

Some of the best foods are made with the fewest tools.

What do penguins use to make pancakes? - Their flippers!

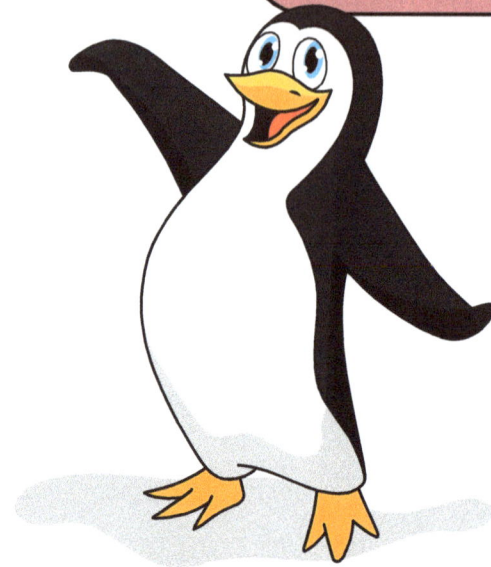

Since you don't have flippers like a penguin, you will need a few things.

Nice to have:

▶ Vegetable peeler, box grater, spatula (for flipping things), knife, wooden spoon for stirring and ladle for sauces, soup, chili...

▶ Large pot, small pot, frying pan and lids.

▶ A few bowls of different sizes for mixing and serving.

▶ Can opener: Best choice is a 'edge-safe' or 'smooth-edge' opener. **Sharp-edge opener: CANS MUST BE OPENED BY AN ADULT!**

▶ Measuring cups, paper towel, cloth towel, scrub brush.

▶ Strainer for draining and steaming veggies.

▶ Brown baking paper and waxed paper: These are GRRR8 choices for our bodies, piggy-bank and our planet.

▶ Reusable storage containers. Empty jars are perfect for storing leftovers, making salad dressing or on the go containers.

▶ Microwave-safe dishes.

▶ Oven mitts keep your hands safe.

▶ Toaster oven, blender, stove.

TRICK Buying used things is GRRR8. You save money and the planet.

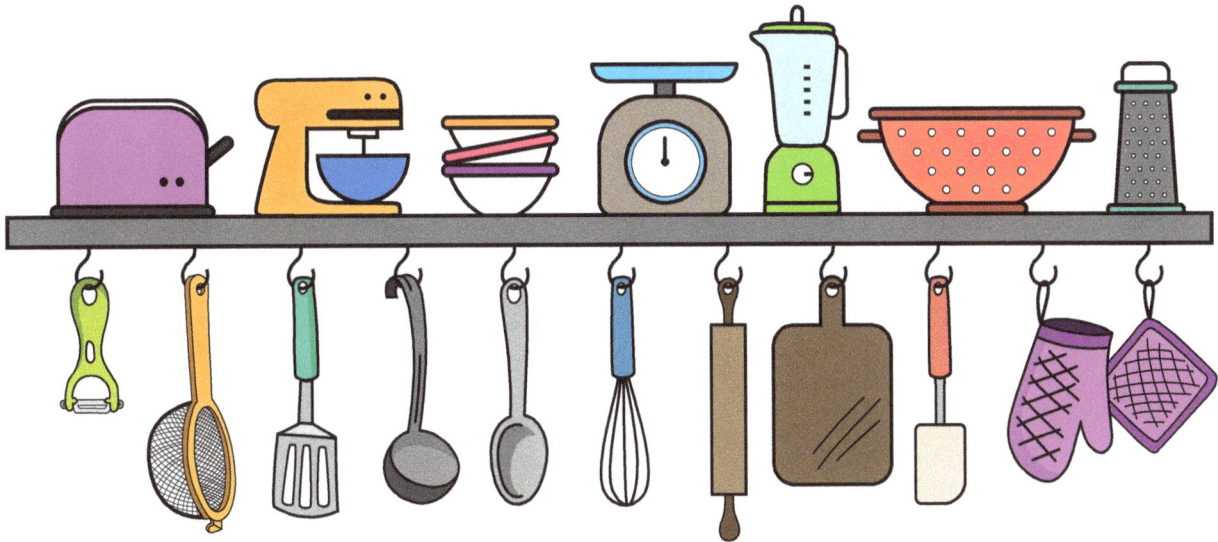

Here are some terms to help you cook like a pro:

BEAT: Stir quickly with a fork or mixer until it is fluffy.

BOIL: A liquid is boiling when it makes noise and has big bubbles on the top.

CHOP: Cut into tiny pieces with a knife.

GRATE: Use a box grater to rub a food item up and down to make it into tiny pieces. This is easier and safer than using a knife.

MASH: Mush or press a food to make a soft mixture.

MINCE: Chop into tiny pieces.

MIX: Stir everything together.

PEEL: Take the outside layer off.

PINCH: Like pinching skin - the amount of spice that fits between your fingers.

PUREE: Think mushy baby food.

SAUTÉ: Quickly cooking at high heat in a little oil on the stovetop.

SLICE: Cut thinly.

SIMMER: A liquid is simmering when you see tiny bubbles on the top.

WHIP: To beat a liquid so strongly it foams (think whipped cream!).

CHECK IT OUT!

MAKE@HOME

Antibacterial Fruit & Veggie Cleaner

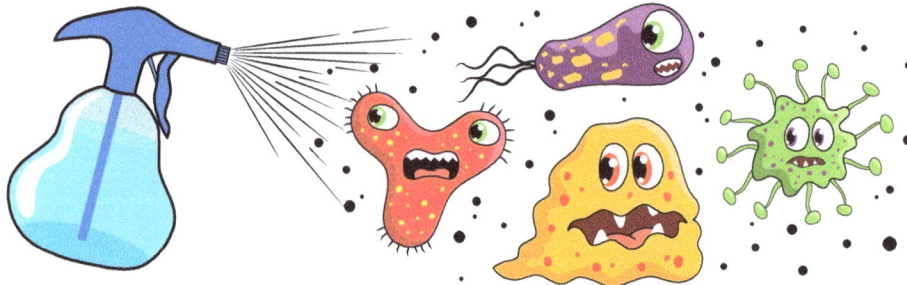

Many vitamins and nutrients are in the skin. Bacteria, pesticides and fungicides can also be on the skin. Most fruits & veggies don't need to be peeled, but do need to be cleaned. Washing with water can reduce 70% of pesticides.

WHAT YOU NEED:

- 1 clean spray bottle
- 8 oz. water
- 1 tbs. white vinegar
- 1 tbs. lemon juice or antibacterial soap (optional)

HOW?

1. Mix the ingredients in the spray bottle
2. Spray fruits and veggies
3. Let sit for 5-10 minutes
4. Rinse with water and let dry.

Vinegar - The Best - Planet Saver - Money Saver - Cleaner

White vinegar is a super cheap antibacterial cleaner for everything. As a natural disinfectant, it can kill germs like salmonella and E. coli.

Mix half water and half white vinegar and a bit of antibacterial soap. Add citrus peels, lavender, ginger or rosemary, if you have some.

Clean everything, from pots, pans, glasses, cutting boards, knives, microwaves, counters and even floors! Add a cup of vinegar to laundry to get rid of stinky smells or for extra-clean clothes.

KITCHEN CLUTTER MATCHING GAME

Connect the words to the kitchen cooking helpers!

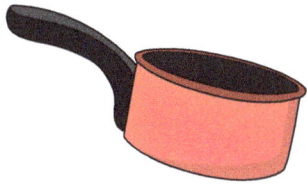

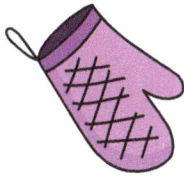

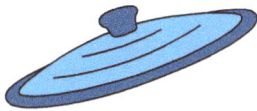

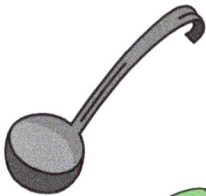

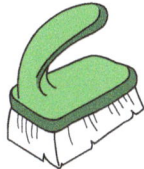

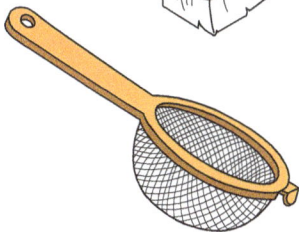

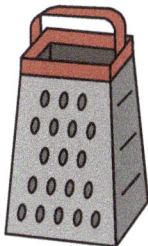

VEGETABLE PEELER

KNIFE

SPATULA

WOODEN SPOON

LADLE

POT

FRYING PAN

LID

MEASURING CUP

STRAINER

METAL SIEVE

SCRUB BRUSH

POT HOLDER

BOX GRATER

SAFE-EDGE CAN OPENER

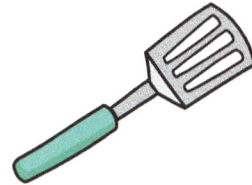

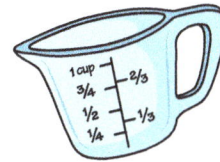

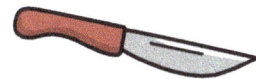

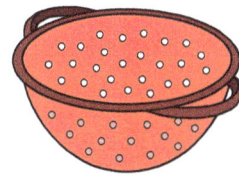

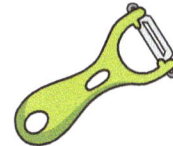

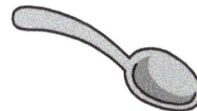

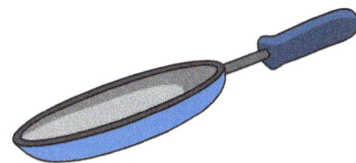

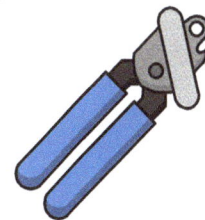

CHECK
IT OUT!

QUICK SNACK TRICKS FOR ON THE GO

Save money and stay satiated until you get home. Keep your heart healthy and happy.

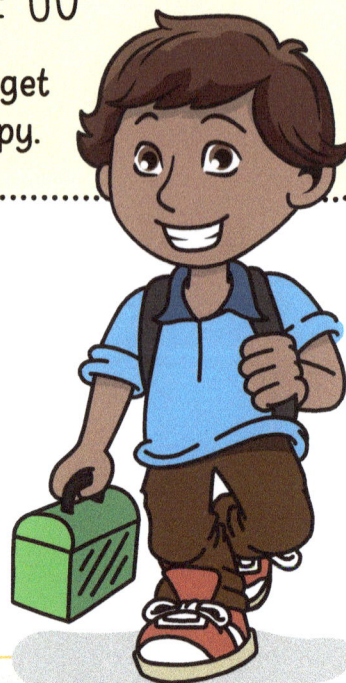

My family has a few tricks to make sure we always manage an affordable Healthy Happy Heart meal, even when we are running short of time.

Make@Home carrot and celery sticks. Keep them in a jar of water in the fridge to grab and go anytime. This snack keeps your teeth happy, too. Crunchy veggies like carrots, peppers, celery sticks, baby tomatoes, and jicama are fun to dunk into easy Make@Home **Happy Healthy Heart** dips. (p. 89)

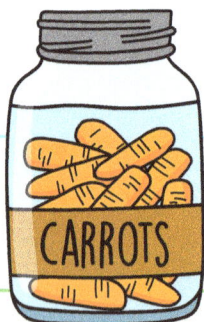

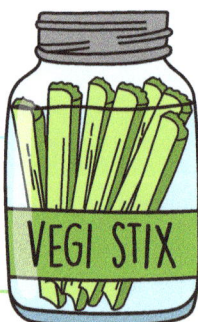

CARROTS

VEGI STIX

Ants on a Log: So easy. Hardest part? Washing the celery.
Fill celery slices with nut butter or cream cheese. Top with oats, nuts or raisins.

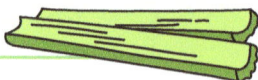

Each weekend:
Keep hard boiled eggs in the fridge for a power snack, breakfast, lunch, or dinner. Each egg has his own packaging, so the earth is happy, too!

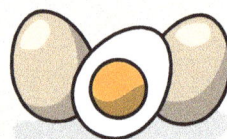

Hard boiled eggs are easy to make. Write the date on them with a pencil. They last about 5 days in the refrigerator. (Check out the egg-cellent recipes on p.92-93)

REMEMBER

ALWAYS READ THE INGREDIENTS before you buy.

These meals take only a few minutes to prepare. They are much cheaper, Happy Heart healthier and use less packaging than pre-made choices. This makes them GRRR8 4 U and the planet.

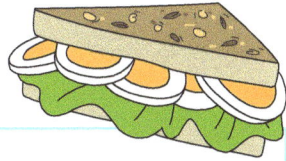

GRRR8 Happy Healthy Heart sandwiches are best with whole grain breads, tortillas or lettuce wraps. (p. 97)

Skip the mayo or ketchup (mostly sugar) for a smear of mustard, yogurt, Healthy Happy Heart bean dip (p.98) or salsa (p.99)

Veggies, leftover egg, beans (p.98), a bit of quick easy chicken (p.108) or cheese make a great wrap.

Oats, water, and anything else, one minute in the microwave. YUM! (p.94)

Go crazy, have fun and listen to your body say, **THANK YOU!**

Apples & bananas are always super snack foods that travel well and taste great. Bananas, apples, a handful of nuts or a few slices of 100% natural cheese = **Fastest Food of All!**

Keep a jar of **Super Sweet Secret Sauce** (p.) in the fridge. Mix into anything you would like a bit sweeter.

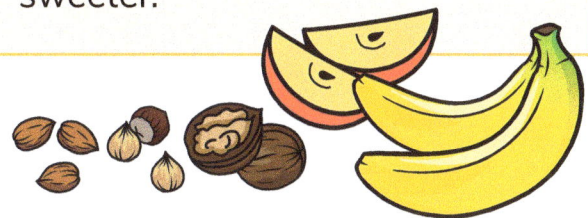

Cheese cubes & apples/nut butter on apples or banana slices takes less time than just about anything.

Plain Yogurt: Add smashed banana, apple, nuts, oats, apple POW!

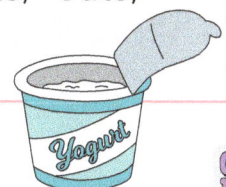

CHECK IT OUT!

SO EASY!

Rad ranch dip/dressing:
- 1/2 cup plain Greek yogurt
- 1 tsp. garlic powder
- 1/2 tsp. onion powder
- 1/2 tsp. dried green herbs like dill, chives, basil, or 1 tsp fresh
- 2 tsp. lemon juice or vinegar Spices to taste (p.102) Optional: 1/4 tsp. honey

Pour in a jar. Close the lid and shake. Add a little water for salad dressing.

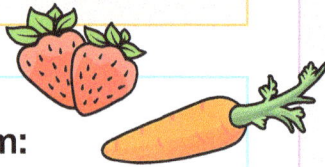

Grab A Bowl of Yum:
Feel like something sweet, cold and crunchy? A bowl of cold carrot, quinoa or fruit salad from the fridge hits the spot. (p.105)

Cool creamy dips: Mix just about anything into plain unsweetened yogurt - spices, mustard, a bit of honey, Super Sweet Secret Sauce, or salsa (p.113). Serve with veggie sticks for Happy Heart party food.

Super Sweet Secret Sauce:
- 1/2 cup dried 100% fruit
- 1/2 cup water or 100% juice
- 1 cup 100% applesauce
- (options: ginger, pumpkin pie spice, or cinnamon)

Soak until the fruit is soft. Cook in the microwave until most of the liquid is gone. Smash with fork. Add applesauce and spices. Cook for 2 minutes. Stir. Cook until it looks like jam or bbq sauce.

Quinoa: This easy **Happy Healthy Heart GRRR8** complete protein is always in our fridge. (p.118) Switch it for rice and pasta. Mix it with fruits or veggies.

Quinoa tacos: Heat a pan with a little oil. Add cooked quinoa, taco spices. Mix well. Cook until crispy. Heat tortillas in a microwave. Serve with sliced crunchy veggies. salsa (p. 113) or yogurt mixed with lime juice or spices. (p.102)
Your heart, brain and bones will LOVE you.

Tricks to eat more fruit and veggies but spend less!
Frozen or canned fruit and veggies are often more affordable than fresh.
They are great for cooking, adding to smoothies or oatmeal.
Be sure to check the label for hidden sugars, salt or fat.

DID YOU KNOW?

Fresh berries are expensive. Frozen berries don't go bad and just a few go a really long way.

Pineapple is a GRRR8 fruit secret packed with vitamins A and C, minerals, antioxidants and fiber. One pineapple gives a lot of servings for the cost.

DID YOU KNOW? 1 serving of pineapple = 18 potato chips or 12 fries.
Pineapple can help with colds, cough, digestion;
strengthen bones, teeth, and muscles; and reduce swelling...

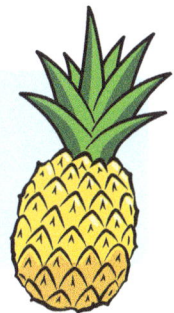

Bananas are super satiating, come perfectly packed and are full of vitamins and minerals. They are healthiest when they get really ripe, start to look yucky AND become cheaper. Smash bananas with a fork and add to cereal, yogurt, nut butter.... just about anything you want sweeter.

Have extra bananas or find some on sale?
Peel, slice and freeze on something flat.
Store the frozen slices in a bag or container.
Enjoy them anytime as ice-cold treats or add
to anything you want to sweeten.

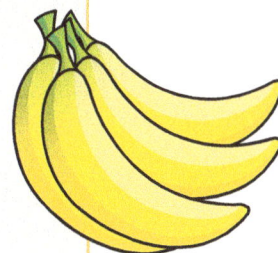

GRRR8 meal in a glass? Smoothies (p. 96), Banana Ice Cream?
Place frozen banana slices in a blender. Blend. Eat. That's it!

CHECK IT OUT!

BAKED APPLES

Servings: 5
1 adult serving: 40 cents

WHAT YOU NEED:

- 3 tbs. coconut sugar, agave or honey
- 4 apples
- 1 cup applesauce
- 2 tsp. cinnamon
- 1 tbs. butter, melted or 100% pumpkin puree
- 1/2 cup plain yogurt
- 1/4 cup water

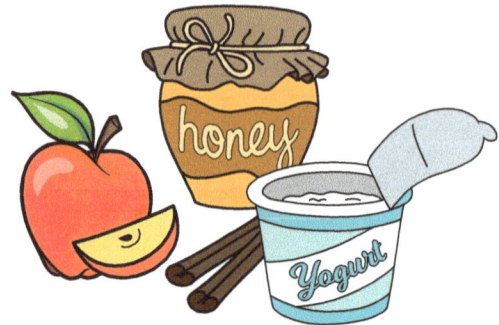

HOW?

With an adult, cut the top off each apple and remove seeds. Melt butter in a microwaveable dish. Add applesauce, cinnamon, and water. Mix well. Place apples, cut side up in the dish.

Spoon a little of the mix in each apple hole and over each apple. Cover with a plate. **Microwave** for 3-5 minutes, until apples are soft. Mix 1 tbs. applesauce with the yogurt in a small bowl.

Serve warm apples with applesauce - yogurt topping.

WARNING!

Careful: Dish will be very hot. Always use a towel or mitt!

EGG—CRACKING TRICKS:

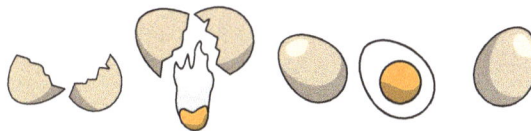

Gently tap the egg on the counter or with the edge of a knife.

Over a small bowl, hold the egg in both hands. Gently push your thumbs into the crack and pull the shell into two parts. Fish out bits of shell that fall in the bowl with a clean finger, spoon or knife. Easy!

Raw egg shells can carry germs! Always wash your hands and anything that touches raw eggs thoroughly with soap and warm water.

HOW TO HARD BOILED EGG

HOW?

Cost per person:
1 egg: 25 cents for a GRRR8 protein deal. ($2.00 per pound, national average.)

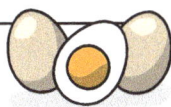

Place eggs in a small pot. Cover with one inch of cold water.
Trick: 1 tsp vinegar in the water keeps eggs from cracking.
Cook over high heat until the water boils.
Boil for one minute, then remove from heat.
Let eggs sit. Hard: 12 minutes. Soft: 9 minutes
Rinse in cool water. Tap on a hard surface and peel away the shell
That's it! Hard-boiled eggs keep in the refrigerator for up to 5 days.

GR8 4 Grab & Go

Write the date on the egg with a pencil. Now, you know when they were cooked. Have fun. Make mini works of art. **TRICK**

WARNING! Boiling water is DANGEROUS! Ask an adult for help!

30 SECOND OMELETTE

Servings: 1
1 adult serving: 0.60 cents

WHAT YOU NEED:

1 egg + 1 tsp. water, beaten with a fork until one color.

HOW?

Heat a frying pan on a medium high heat. Rub the pan with a little butter or oil. Add the egg, tipping the egg mixture until the pan is coated with a thin yellow layer.

On half the omelet, sprinkle with anything else you are adding. Tip: Heat **extras like chopped veggies, beans, potato, quinoa** in the micro. **Cheeses, parsley, cilantro or salsas** can either go inside or on top. Fold the empty side on top. Slide onto a plate and ta-daa! Eat with a fork, wrap it in a tortilla or in a whole grain bread cut in 1/2.

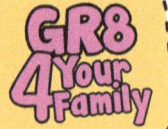

GR8 4 Your Family

SUNSHINE EGGS

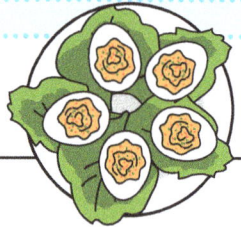

Servings: 4
1 adult serving: 35 cents

WHAT YOU NEED:

- 4 hard cooked peeled eggs
- 1 tbs. plain greek yogurt (no added sugar)

Extras: squeeze of lemon, dried spices, chopped basil, parsley, green onion, cilantro, 1 tbs. mustard, salsa (p. 102)...

HOW?

Hold the egg long side down. Slice in half. Mix in any 'extras'. Put the yolks (the yellow balls), yogurt and any of the extras into a bowl. Smash with a fork. Refill the holes with spoonfuls of the yolk mix or put yolks in a small plastic bag and cut a little bit off the corner. Place them on a plate. The QR code shows you how you can dye them. Make Art! Top with a sprinkle of spice, a drop of mustard, a parsley leaf, a slice of olive or create happy faces!

BIG BROTHER'S YUMMIEST GOOD-ANY-TIME OATMEAL TREAT

1 adult power packed meal: 60 cents

WHAT YOU NEED:

- 1/3 cup oats
- 3/4 cup water, powdered, plant-based or dairy milk

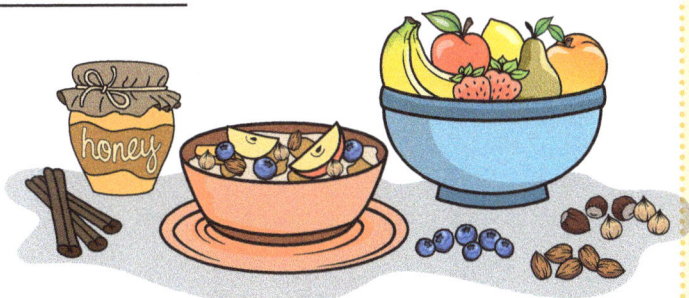

Extras: A scoop of plain yogurt, chopped banana or apple, a few raisins, frozen berries or chopped nuts, a sprinkle of cinnamon, 1 tbs. of nut butter, pumpkin or a drizzle of honey. The combinations are endlessly delicious.

HOW?

Put everything in a microwaveable bowl. Microwave for 1 minute.
Careful: Bowl will be very hot - always use a towel or mitt!
Stir and microwave again for another minute. After you have done this a few times you will know exactly how long it takes to cook a bowl of oatmeal in your microwave. All microwaves are different. Stir. Top with more yummy extras. Dig into the best meal ever!

TRICK

Make a big bowl of oatmeal and store it in the fridge. Just scoop out a portion and reheat for an instant meal or snack. Fill a bunch of single-serve microwave-safe jars. Add your favorite toppings. All you do is grab, take off the lid and in the microwave it goes. BAMM!

CHECK IT OUT!

AUNTIE'S AMAZING MILK (HORCHATA)

Servings: 8
1 adult serving: 25 cents

It takes about 5 minutes to make your very own 'milk'.

Kitchen tools: Blender, bowl, a mesh sieve or a thin piece of clean cloth. This also works with any kind of nuts for homemade nut milk.

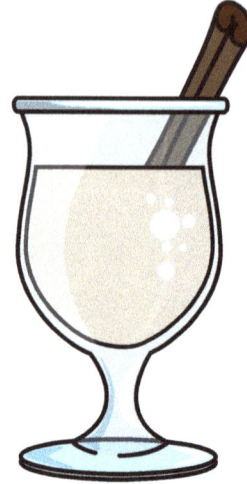

WHAT YOU NEED:

- 6 cups water
- 1 cup rice or raw oats.
- 1 cup unsweetened plant or dairy "milk"

Extras: a few pitted dates, prunes, 1/2 tsp. vanilla, 2 whole cinnamon sticks or 1/2 tsp. powdered cinnamon, 1/2 cup powdered milk or unsweetened cocoa powder for chocolate "milk"

HOW?

Put rice or oats, cinnamon, and water in a blender and let everything soak for about 20 minutes.
Blend until smooth. Super yummy: let it rest in the fridge for a few hours or overnight.
Pour through a sieve.
Store horchata in a glass jar in the refrigerator for up to 5 days.
Some bits will settle at the bottom. That is ok.

ENJOY!

SUPER SATIATING SMOOTHY MEAL

Servings: 2
1 adult serving: 50 cents

WHAT YOU NEED:

- 1 cup 'milk' (fresh, powdered or homemade), horchata or yogurt
- 1 banana sliced, fresh or frozen

HOW?

Put everything in a blender. Cover tightly. Blend until smooth.
Stay fueled for hours.

Extras: 1 pitted date, 1/2 cup fruit-fresh, frozen or 100% canned, 1 tbs. nut butter, nuts, 1/2 cup spinach (no taste+great color), ice

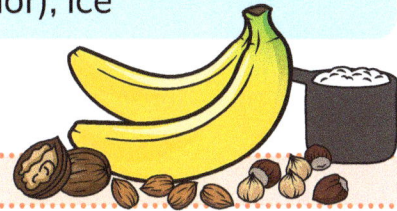

BANANA OAT POWER BALLS

Servings: 8
1 adult serving: 30 cents

WHAT YOU NEED:

- 2 1/2 cups uncooked oats (not steel-cut)
- 1 tsp. ground cinnamon
- 2 tbs. coconut sugar, agave syrup or honey
- 1/4 cup nut butter
- 2 ripe mashed bananas (about 1 c.)

Extras: handful of raisins, chopped nuts, chocolate chips, seeds, pumpkin, or mix it up. ½ cups unsweetened shredded coconut for rolling

HOW?

Mix oats and cinnamon in a large bowl. Add mashed banana, nut butter, sweetener and any of the options. Stir until ingredients are well blended.
Shape into 24 1-inch balls. You can roll them in shredded coconut. Store leftovers in the refrigerator, covered.

CHECK IT OUT!

BEAN AND CHEESE BURRITO

Servings: 10
1 adult serving: 60 cents
1/2 burrito = 1 kid portion

WHAT YOU NEED:

- 1 15 oz. can vegetarian refried beans or whole beans
- 10 full grain burrito size tortillas
- 1/2 cup salsa (p. 102)
- 1 small onion, chopped
- 1/2 cup cottage cheese
- 1/2 cup shredded cheese

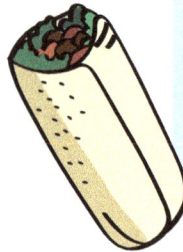

Extras: cooked: rice, quinoa, potato, cooked meat or egg, fresh chopped vegetables: spinach, lettuce, tomato, peppers, cilantro, corn (p. 102)

HOW?

Mix everything together in a bowl and any extras, you like.
Make a rectangle in the middle of each wrap with an equal amount of the mixture.

Fold the top and bottom flaps in over the filling. Fold in the sides. Place the bundles, fold-sides down, in a microwaveable dish. Microwave on high for 2-6 minute, depending on how many you are heating and your microwave. Use a cloth when removing the hot dish from the microwave. Wrap in foil or waxed paper. Store in the fridge or freeze.

Serve with Party Salsa Fresca, sour cream, more veggies, or fruit.

REMEMBER

**If you don't have an 'edge-safe can opener:
CANS MUST BE OPENED BY AN ADULT!**

FUNNY FACE SANDWICHES

1 adult serving:
60-80 cents

WHAT YOU NEED:

- One slice of whole grain bread.
- 100% nut butter, bean spread, cottage or cream cheese
- Fresh or dried fruit, veggies, seeds or nuts.

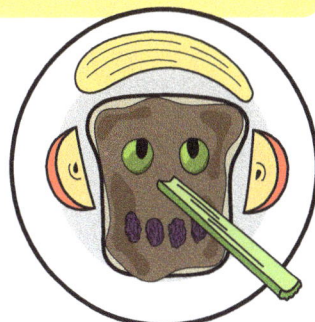

HOW?

Spread a thin layer of your favorite Happy Heart spread.
Create a face. Use seeds, nuts, olives or slices of different veggies or fruits. Grated carrots, parsley, cilantro or celery leaves make great hair. Use raisins for a very scary smile.

BUBBA'S BEST BEAN SPREAD FOR WRAPS, DIP, OR DRESSING

1 adult serving:
30 cents

WHAT YOU NEED:

- 1 15-ounce can beans or lentils, drained but save the liquid
- 1 clove garlic, peeled or 1/8 tsp. garlic powder
- 3 tbs. **Happy Healthy Heart** oil
- 2 tbs. lemon juice or vinegar

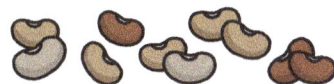

Extras: pepper (p. 102), paprika cumin, 3 stems parsley or cilantro

HOW?

Put everything in a blender with 1/2 the liquid from the bean can. Blend until smooth and creamy.
Add water, spoon by spoon until it looks like baby food.
Eat it straight as a dip with carrots, celery, jicama sticks, lettuce leaves, or whole-grain crackers. Super Salad Dressing: add a little vinegar and water or apple juice.

CHECK IT OUT!

PARTY SALSA FRESCA

Servings: 8
1 adult serving: 25 cents

Help prepare this great dish.
Draw a line for each ingredient amount. Label and color each section.
It couldn't be easier or healthier.

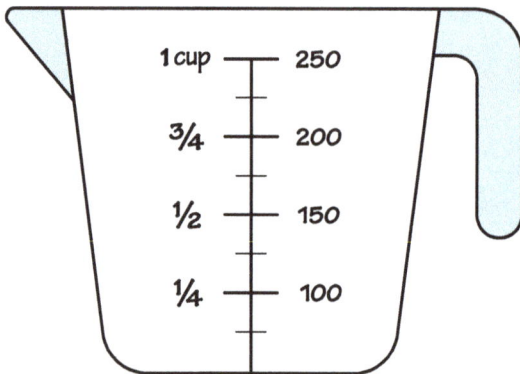

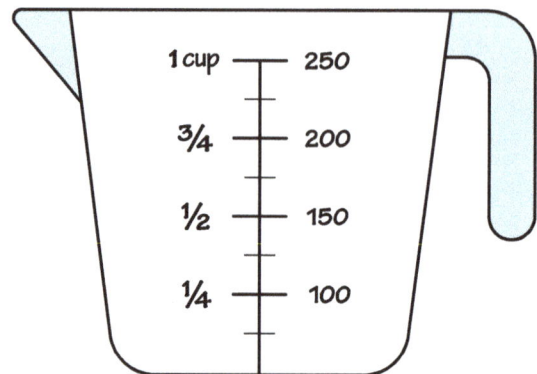

1 cup — 250	1 cup — 250
¾ — 200	¾ — 200
½ — 150	½ — 150
¼ — 100	¼ — 100

WHAT YOU NEED:

- 1½ cups chopped tomatoes
- ¼ cup chopped white onion
- ¼ cup chopped cilantro
- 1 tbs. lime juice, to taste
- Spices to taste (p. 102)

Option: Add 1 cup chopped pineapple or a jalapeno pepper, seeds removed and chopped

HOW?

Mix everything in a bowl. Stir and gobble up!
Even easier Salsa? No need to chop, just dump all the above in a blender. Use vinegar instead of lime juice. Yum!!

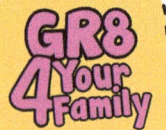

GR8 4 Your Family

TRICK Don't wait for a party to make this at home. Keep these super delicious, healthy fiber and vitamin-packed snacks in the fridge. Try them on eggs, potatoes, beans, rice or in quinoa tacos. Mix some in yogurt for a creamy dip or Happy Healthy Heart salad dressing.

CHECK IT OUT!

GRRR8 GRATED CARROT SALAD

Servings: 4
1 adult serving: 25 cents

WHAT YOU NEED:

- 1 pound carrots, peeled and grated
- 1 tbs. **Happy Healthy Heart** oil
- 1/4 cup sugar-free orange, apple or other juice

Extras: quinoa, pineapple, raisins, celery, apple, chopped mint, parsley, nuts, beans, chickpeas, cinnamon...

HOW?

Place everything in a bowl and stir. That's it! So easy.

EASIEST AND MOST DIVINE TOMATO SAUCE

Servings: 6-8
1 adult serving: 26 cents

Use this on quinoa or pasta. Make your own pizza. Cook an egg in it. Let your imagination fly.

WHAT YOU NEED:

- 1 large 28-oz can of diced tomatoes
- 1/4 c. **Happy Healthy Heart** oil
- ½ tsp. garlic powder or 2 cloves peeled and cut in half.
- 1 small onion, grated or chopped
- 1 small carrot, grated
- Spices to taste (p. 102)

HOW?

Heat oil in a pan or pot. Pour everything into a pan or pot and heat on medium high. Cook for about 10 minutes on low heat. The longer it cooks, the thicker it gets. Take off heat. Once it cools, dig in! Store in the fridge for up to one week or freeze. I bet it doesn't last that long!

CHECK IT OUT!

THREE SISTERS X FOUR

Servings: 10
1 adult serving: 30 cents

Three Sisters: corn, beans and squash
symbolize family and community for America's First People.
Planted together, beans climb up the tall corn stalks. As the beans
grow, they add nitrogen to the soil to feed the squash. Big squash
leaves shade the soil, keeping out weeds and saving water.
Three Sisters, like all of us, grow best when we help each other.

WHAT YOU NEED:

- 1 15-oz can beans, drained
- 1 15-oz can sweet corn, drained
- 1 zucchini or squash, grated
- 1 bunch cilantro, chopped
- 2 tbs. lime, lemon juice or vinegar
- 2 tbs. Happy Heart oil
- Spices to taste (p. 102)

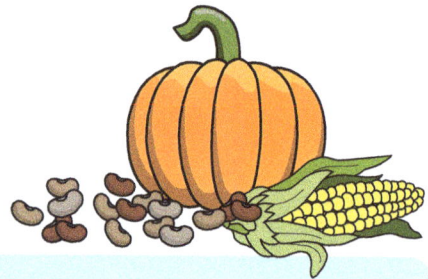

Extras: quinoa, rice, salsa, chopped jalapeño-seeds carefully removed, potato, grated or cottage cheese

HOW?

Mix everything together in a bowl. That's it!

#1: Make it a meal: Add a side of greens, rice, quinoa, lentils, or potato.

#2: Make a sandwich wrap: Spoon some on a tortilla with any of the extras. Fold up the bottom flap and give it a roll.

#3: Taco: Heat in a microwave or on the stove. Place in a warm tortilla. Top with any of the extras.

#4: Soup: Heat in a pot with 4 cups of vegetable broth. (Skip the lemon or vinegar.)

REMEMBER If you don't have an 'edge-safe can opener: CANS MUST BE OPENED BY AN ADULT!

SUPER SIDE OF SPINACH

WHAT YOU NEED:

- 12-oz spinach, fresh or frozen
- 2 tbls. **Happy Healthy Heart** oil
- 2 tsp. garlic powder
- Spices to taste (p. 102)

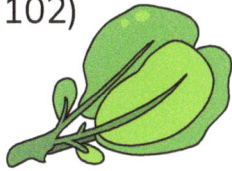

HOW?

Heat 1/4 cup of water in a large pan on medium-high heat.

Add the garlic, oil, any other spices, beans or peas, if using.

Add the spinach and mix until the leaves are warm but a bright, shiny green color. This only takes a few minutes. Remove from heat.

Add any other extras or toppings.

Servings: 4
1 adult serving: 40 cents
With cheese and beans:
8 servings - 40 cents a serving

Extras: 1 12-oz. bag frozen peas, 1 15-oz. can beans, drained (Some say black-eyed peas bring good-luck!), 1 cup small curd cottage cheese, grated cheese, salsa...

Extra Toppings:
4 oz. chopped roasted peanuts, diced raw onions, tomatoes

TRICK

Just say no when a recipe says to add salt. Squeeze a little fruit juice, grate some citrus peel, add a spoon of salsa or mustard or add a splash of vinegar instead of salt for a yummier yum.

Choose dried spices like onion, garlic, mint, dill, pepper or oregano from the bulk section at the store. They are much cheaper. You can buy a small amount and try lots of better flavor combinations

CHECK IT OUT!

GRRR8 GREEN SPINACH PASTA

Servings: 8
1 adult serving: 15-30 cents

WHAT YOU NEED:

- 6 oz. spinach, fresh or frozen (about 3/4 c. blended)
- 3 tbs. **Happy Healthy Heart** oil
- 2¼ cups flour plus extra for dusting

Make different colored pasta. Use 3/4 c. pumpkin, sweet potato or squash puree, pea, tomato paste and herbs, carrot or beet juice...

HOW?

Food processor: Blitz spinach and oil. Add flour until a ball of dough forms.

Blender: Blend spinach and oil. Make a hole in the middle of the flour in a bowl. Pour in spinach and mix. Dough should feel like playdough, not sticky. Add a little flour if needed.

Roll out on a floured counter and cut into shapes with cookie cutters. Roll up and cut with a knife into strips or shape into skinny, thin snakes or green beans. Cook fresh, freeze or dry overnight.

Cook in boiling water for 5 minutes, if fresh, 8 to 10 minutes, if dry and depending on thickness.

Ask an adult to drain. Save a cupful of cooking water to add to pasta sauce, as needed.

Watch this link for a great sauce. You can substitute butternut squash with one can of 100% pure pumpkin.

CHECK IT OUT!

BB AND SIS'S SMASHED POTATOES

Servings: 5
1 adult serving: 80 cents

WHAT YOU NEED:

Extra: 1 tbs. of butter

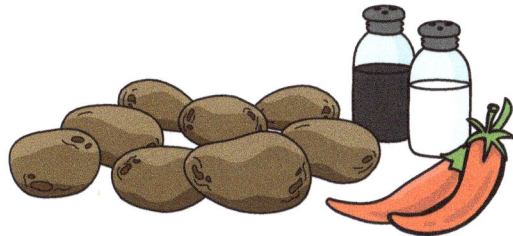

- 4 medium yukon gold or russet potatoes, washed and cut in half.
- Water
- Add to taste: Spices (p. 102) or powdered milk

HOW?

Place potato pieces in a pot of cold water. Cover. Heat on high. Once the water starts to boil, turn the heat down to medium to simmer. Remove the lid.

WARNING! WITH AN ADULT! Drain the water.

Potatoes are cooked when they poke easily with a fork.

Save about one cup of the hot potato water for mashing into the potatoes. If adding dried milk, add milk to hot potato water, according to directions.

Smash the potatoes with a potato masher or fork. Add butter and spices. Keep adding hot potato water to the pot until they are perfect.

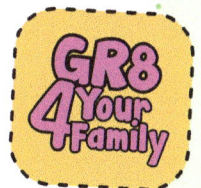

GR8 4 Your Family

PUMPKIN PUDDING

Servings: 10
1 adult serving: 36 cents

WHAT YOU NEED:

- 1 can 100% pure pumpkin
- 1/2 cup apple sauce
- 3 cups water
- 1 cup cornmeal or polenta
- 1 tbs. butter (optional)
- 1/2 tsp. ground cinnamon
- 1 cup small curd cottage cheese
- 2 cups milk

Topping: A spoon of yogurt sweetened with banana slices, a dust of cinnamon or Secret Sauce (p.89).

HOW?

Bring pumpkin, apple sauce and water to a boil in a saucepan over medium heat. Keep stirring

On low heat, stir in polenta or cornmeal and cinnamon. Stir often for about 15 minutes.

Add the cottage cheese, milk and butter.

Cook on low for about 5 more minutes. Keep stirring.

Serve in bowls or glasses.

DID YOU KNOW?

Pumpkin and squash are packed with Happy Healthy Heart fiber, vitamins, minerals and antioxidants. Buy after Thanksgiving, when cans go on sale.
Did you know you can swap canned 100% pumpkin for eggs, oil and butter?

1 egg =	1 tbs. oil =	1 tbs. butter =
1/4 c pumpkin	1 tbs. pumpkin	1 tbs. pumpkin

PUMPKIN CHILI

Servings: 12
1 adult serving: 75 cents.

WHAT YOU NEED:

- 2 tbs. **Happy Healthy Heart** oil
- 1 c. chopped white onion
- 1 tbs. chopped garlic or 1 tsp. garlic powder
- 1 tbs. chili powder
- 2 c. vegetable stock
- 1 can (15 oz.) diced tomatoes
- 1 can (15 oz.) white beans, drained
- 1 can (15 oz.) chickpeas, drained
- 1 bag (10 oz.) frozen diced butternut squash
- 1 can (15 oz.) 100% pure pumpkin puree
- Spices to taste (p. 102)

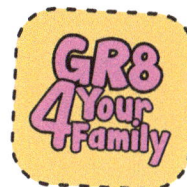

GR8
4 Your
Family

Toppings: plain yogurt, grated cheese, chopped cucumber...

HOW?

Heat on medium everything in a large pot.

Cook onion and garlic until soft. Add chili powder.

Stir and cook 2-3 minutes; add stock. Bring to a low simmer, then add tomatoes, beans, chickpeas, butternut squash and pumpkin.

Turn heat to low. Stir, so it doesn't burn. Cook for 30-40 minutes.

FAST AND EASY VEGETABLE SOUP

Servings: 8
1 adult serving: 45 cents

WHAT YOU NEED:

- 1 12-oz bag frozen veggies: cauliflower, cauliflower/broccoli, carrots, carrot/pea, zucchini blend, or butternut squash or a can of pumpkin puree.
- 1 large onion, chopped
- 2 garlic cloves, crushed
- 2 cups water
- 2 cups unsweetened 'milk'
- Spices to taste (p. 102)

Extras: frozen corn, peas, chopped greens, lemon cottage or grated cheese.

HOW?

Place onion, garlic, veggies and water in a pot. Cook on high heat until it boils. Lower heat and simmer for about 10 minutes or until everything is soft. Remove from heat.

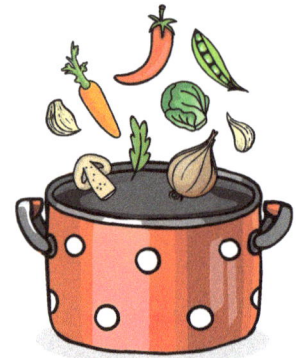

WARNING!

Let cool for about 30 minutes. Blending hot solids and liquids is very dangerous. It can explode and cause burns.

Carefully, scoop the vegetables out and place in a blender. Put a towel over the lid and press the lid tight. Blend with some of the cooking liquid. Pour back into the pot.

Add "milk", spices and any extras you like. Reheat on medium. Do not let soup boil once the milk is added.

Serve in bowls. Sprinkle with chopped greens, cheese, spices, a squeeze of lemon...

CRAZY QUICK INSTANT CHICKEN GREAT FOR EVERYTHING

Servings: 6
1 adult serving: 80 cents

With this in the fridge you are only minutes away from the super fastest of fast foods. Make sandwiches and wraps in a snap. Throw this powerful protein on top of soup, salad, tacos or noodles.

Eat as-is or with mustard, Healthy Happy Heart sauces, or a little hot sauce and honey. Yummy hot, room temperature, or cold, whole, sliced or shredded with a fork.

WHAT YOU NEED:

- Skinless chicken pieces
- Water

Extras: vegetable broth, lemon pieces, dry spices, jar of salsa, ginger, chilis, onion, garlic...

HOW?

Place skinless chicken pieces in a pot. Add anything else you like. Cover with warm water so the water level is about one inch higher. Bring to a boil over medium-high heat. Then, cover and reduce heat for a low simmer.
Chicken is done when there is no pink inside the thickest part (20-30 minutes depending on size, thickness and bones).
For frozen chicken, add about 10 minutes to the cooking time.
Remove the chicken and place on a plate or clean cutting board.
Strain and save liquid for making quinoa, soups, rice, or pasta either in the fridge (up to 4 days) or freeze. Store leftover chicken in the refrigerator for up to 4 days or freeze.

SHAKE AND BAKE NUGGETS — CAULIFLOWER OR CHICKEN

Servings: 8
1 adult serving:
- Chicken: 90 cents
- Cauliflower: 60 cents

Faster, yummier and costs less than a bag of frozen nuggets.

WHAT YOU NEED:

- 2 pounds skinless chicken meat or 1 cauliflower head, pre-cooked*
- 1 cup flour in a paper or sealable plastic bag or plate
- 1 large egg broken into a sealable plastic bag or bowl
- 1 cup bread crumbs or crushed cornflakes* in a paper or sealable plastic bag or plate
- Spices to taste (p. 102)

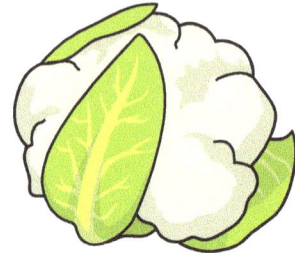

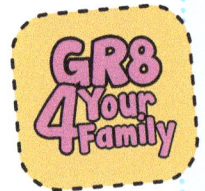

HOW?

You can add flavors like grated cheese, sesame seeds, dried spices or grated lemon peel to any of the bags or add mustard to the egg. Mix up the egg with a fork.

Use a plastic cutting board. Cut chicken into nugget-sized pieces about 1-inch wide. Sprinkle with spices.

1-2-3 Coat:

Drop the pieces into the flour bag. Close the bag and shake, coating each piece. Gently shake off any extra flour.

Move the pieces to the egg bag or bowl. Smoosh the nuggets around until coated.

Dump the eggy pieces into the bread crumbs. Close the bag and shake. Put nuggets on a plate and flatten with your hand.

Oven or air fryer: Heat oven to 350°. Line a cookie sheet with baking paper or foil. Coat lightly with **Happy Healthy Heart** oil. Space nuggets on cookie sheet. Bake for about 7 minutes on each side. Cook what you need or freeze flat on a tray. Once frozen, store in a tub or sealable bags. Cooked chicken has no pink inside.

Stovetop: Heat a frying pan with a few teaspoons of oil on medium high heat. Add nuggets to the pan. Don't crowd them. Give them space. Cook on each side until golden, about five minutes. Flip with a fork or tongs.

*How to crush cornflakes: Pour cornflakes in a bag. Smash with something heavy - or your fist! (or use a blender)

*How to pre-cook cauliflower: Break into 2-3 flowers. Add pieces, 1 tsp. water, and any spices into a microwaveable bowl.
Cook for 2 minute. Let cool.

PERFECT FLUFFY QUINOA

Servings: 4
1 adult serving: 80 cents

WHAT YOU NEED:

- 1 cup uncooked quinoa
- 2 cups water or broth

Extras: Spices (p. 102), grated veggies, beans, salsa, pineapple, just about anything! Or try the yummy muffins in the link below.

HOW?

Rinse quinoa with cold water in a bowl. Carefully pour out water and rinse again.

Put quinoa and liquid in a pot and bring to a boil. Once boiling, reduce heat to low, cover and let simmer for 15 minutes. Remove from heat. Let it rest for 10 minutes. NO PEEKING! Fluff with a fork.

FROZEN FRUIT YOGURT

Servings: 8
1 adult serving: 30 cents

WHAT YOU NEED:

- 1 cup frozen fruit
- 1 frozen banana
- 2 cups Greek yogurt
- **Options:** dried chopped pitted dates or plums for extra sweetness

Toppings: chopped fruit, nuts, toasted coconut, a sprinkle of cinnamon.

HOW?

Put everything in a food processor or blender. Blend until smooth and creamy. Scoop into bowls or freeze in a container with a lid.

APPLE "DONUTS"

Servings: 2
1 adult serving: 70 cents

WHAT YOU NEED:

- 1 apple
- 100% nut butter or cream cheese

Toppings: chopped fruit, nuts, toasted coconut, a sprinkle of cinnamon, a drizzle of melted chocolate

HOW?

Apple rings: Slice the apple across into 4. Remove the apple core and seeds with a small knife. Cover each ring with spread. Sprinkle with your favorite toppings.

NUT BUTTER CRISPY TREATS

Servings: 30
1 ball: 10 cents

WHAT YOU NEED:

- • 1 cup sugar free creamy nut butter
- • 1 cup sugar free crispy rice cereal
- • 1 raw oats
- • 1/2 cup raisins
- 1/2 cup Secret Sauce or 4 smashed soaked prunes* (p.89)

Toppings: chopped fruit, nuts, toasted coconut, a sprinkle of cinnamon.

HOW?

Line a tray with baking or wax paper. Microwave prunes/sauce and nut butter in a large microwave safe bowl for 20 seconds on medium. Stir. Add everything else and mix thoroughly. Chill for 20 minutes. Make bite-sized balls using two spoons. Roll in any of the toppings. Chill balls in the refrigerator for one hour. Store covered in the fridge.
*Cook in microwave until kind of sticky

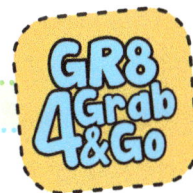

GR8
4 Grab
&Go

MADE@HOME FRUIT POPSICLE:

HOW?

Cut soft fruit into tiny pieces. Place in popsicle molds or small paper cups. Pour in horchata or juice flavored water. Add popsicle sticks and freeze.

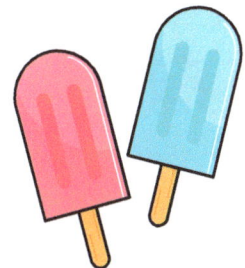

ONE LAST THING TO THINK ABOUT– SALT

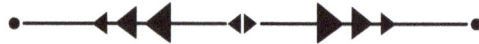

Doctors and scientists are very worried because kids- like adults- eat too much salt.

Why does this matter?
Too much salt can cause heart, kidney, bladder, bone or breathing problems.

School kids need about 1800 milligrams of salt (sodium chloride or NaCl) each day for the body to stay balanced. However, most kids get between 3300-5000 milligrams each day. The older kids get, the more salt they eat. Most of the salt comes from pre-made and restaurant foods, like snacks, burgers, pizza, fries and sliced luncheon meats. Just one fast food kid's meal has about 1500 milligrams or sodium.

Make your body happier by switching fruit and yogurt for chips or chicken or tuna for sliced deli meat.

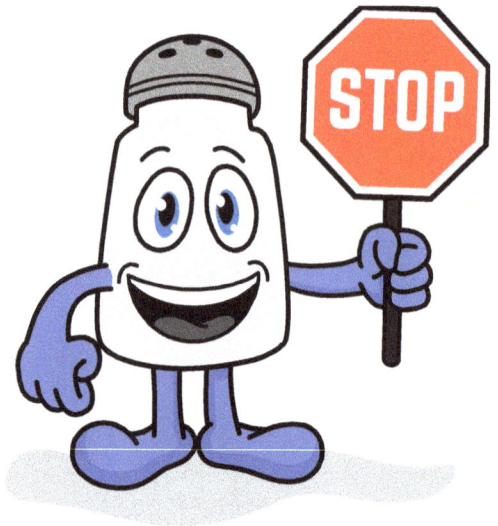

TRY THIS EXPERIMENT

Put 2 slices of cucumber or tomato on two plates. Sprinkle one slice with salt. Let rest for one hour.
- Was there a change? What happened?
- Do you think the same will happen to your bones or organs?

REMEMBER

Always check labels for hidden salt and sugars. Packaging can be very sneaky. It may say it is full of something very healthy on the package. It may have only the tiniest amount, but costs more because people think it is "healthy".

THINGS I WANT TO REMEMBER

Write notes or draw pictures of just about anything you
have learned that you find interesting.

TAKE A TRIP AROUND THE WORLD

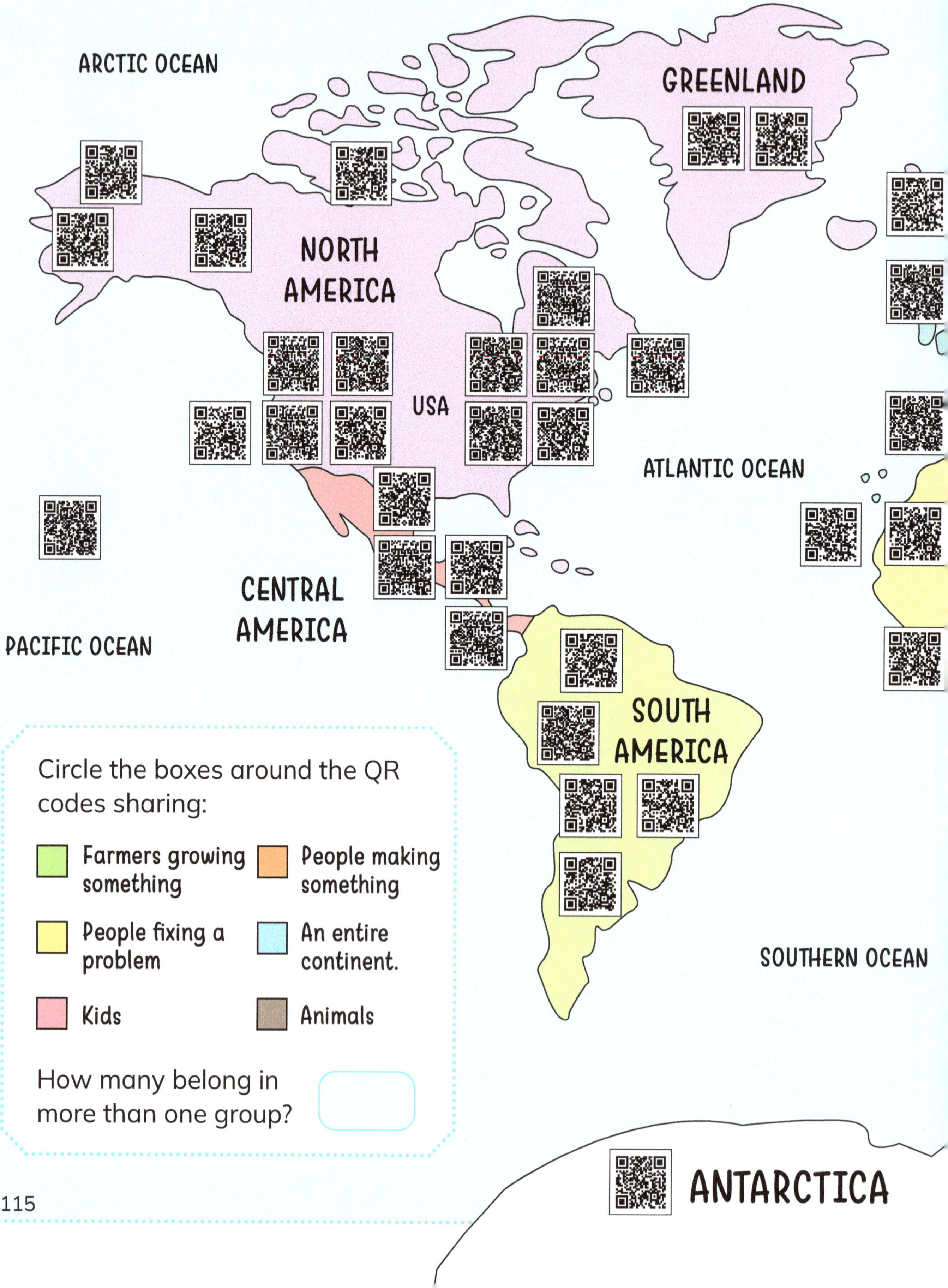

ARCTIC OCEAN

GREENLAND

NORTH AMERICA

USA

ATLANTIC OCEAN

CENTRAL AMERICA

PACIFIC OCEAN

SOUTH AMERICA

SOUTHERN OCEAN

Circle the boxes around the QR codes sharing:

- 🟩 Farmers growing something
- 🟧 People making something
- 🟨 People fixing a problem
- 🟦 An entire continent.
- 🟥 Kids
- ⬜ Animals

How many belong in more than one group?

ANTARCTICA

ARCTIC OCEAN

EUROPE

ASIA

AFRICA

PACIFIC OCEAN

INDIAN OCEAN

AUSTRALIA

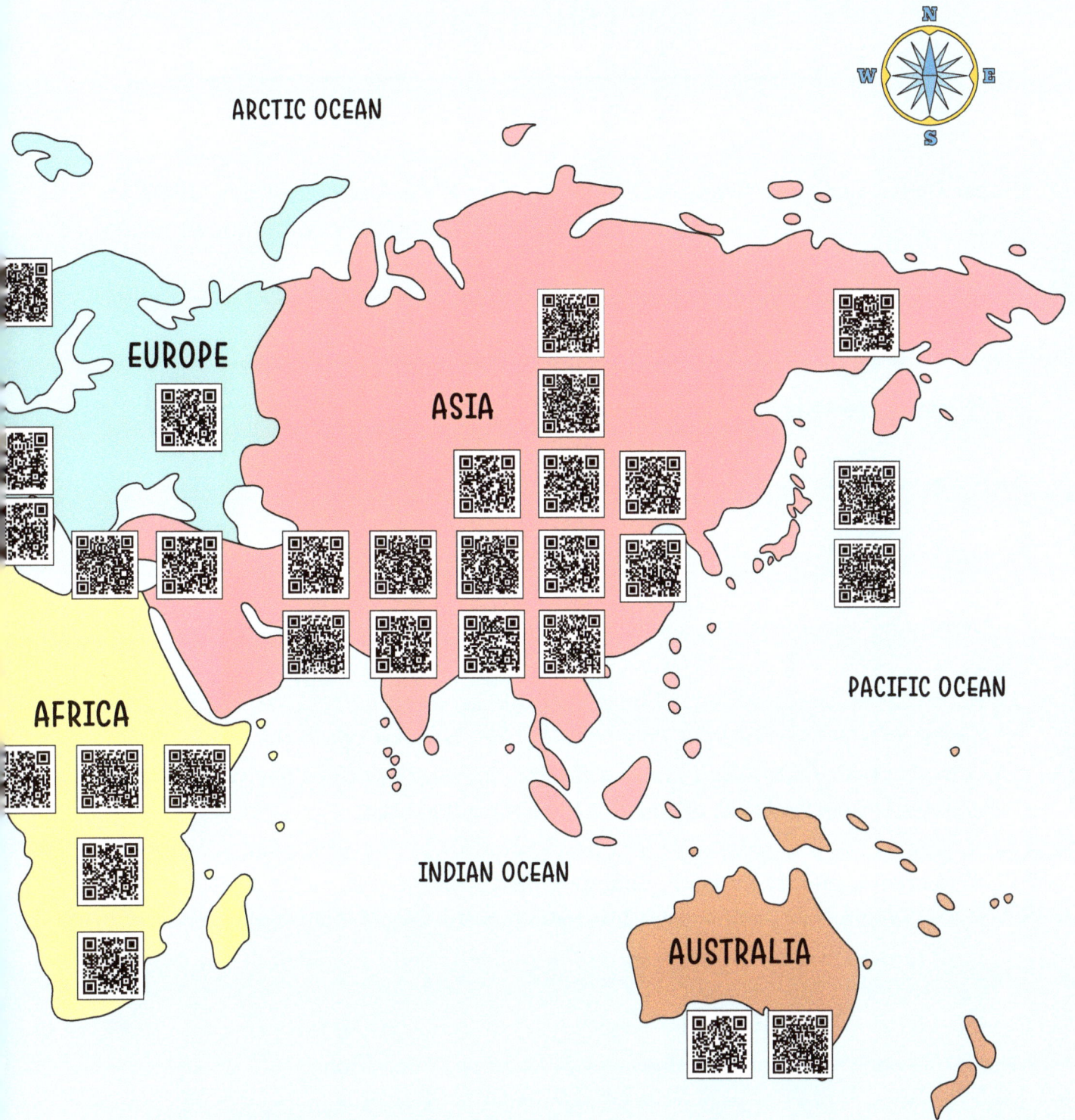

More to explore:

ONLY SCIENTISTS LIVE HERE. NOTHING GROWS ON ICE.

DEAR HOME TEAM

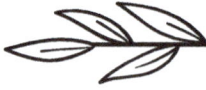

GAME PLAN

Super Me is a fun interactive workbook focusing on whole-health literacy & **STEMM***.

* **S**CIENCE, **T**ECHNOLOGY, **E**NGINEERING, **M**ATH AND **M**EDICINE)

Super Me explains how success in school and growing strong bodies has lots to do with the smallest everyday choices we make.

Life patterns created now, help kids re-imagine their future.

Here are some tips:

- Ask your child to complete 2 pages of Super Me a day or 1 chapter each week.

- Watch the videos linked throughout the book together. Ask: What did you learn?

- Read the Super Me Revolution Challenge (p.46) section together. Ask your family to pledge to take the challenge. This gets your kids cooking, planning meals, helping with shopping, researching, reading, discussing healthy choices and writing. Start with the recipes and links provided in the back of the book.

- Give them a budget for each meal they plan. Ask them to make a list and give you an approximate total cost. (Give them a break on the little things like oil and spices.) Have them look up prices on the website where you shop or any big box store, entering your zip code.

The inside back cover has sites and links full of helpful information.

Have a great Healthy Heart adventure,

Adi

Educational / Motivational QR Links Supporting the National Challenge to Build Healthy Communities

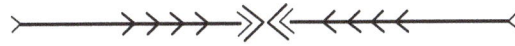

———— >>>> >|<← <<<< ————

Never Give Up, Believe in Yourself / Mulligan Brothers
Introduction to Tools for Supporting Emotional Wellbeing in Children and Youth / *The National Academies of Sciences, Engineering, and Medicine*
2 Water Walk /WaterAid
6 What Does Soda Do to Your Body? / *It's AumSum Time*
7 What Would Happen If You Didn't Drink Water?
/ *Mia Naamuli TED-ED*
8 Fueling My Healthy Life / *MyPlate.gov*
9 What is Metabolism? / *Van Andel Institute*
10 Wellbeing for Children: Healthy Habits / *Elementary & Middle School Resources*
11 Kids Learn Why Bees Are Awesome / *National Geographic*
12 Why Do Bees Build Hexagonal Honeycombs? / *BBC*
13 Quinoa History and Nutrition - Superfoods
/ *WatchSuperFoods*
14 How to Make Overnight Oats / Quaker
15 Microwave Coee Cup Scramble / *Incredible Egg*
16 What Comes from an Egg? / *Planet Nutshell*
18 How to Measure - For Kids / *Cooking with Kids, Inc*
19 The Color Wheel / *Ehullquist*
22 Urban SNAP-Ed Easy, Tasty, and Aordable Recipe: Hummus / *Alabama Extension*
23 Understanding Fibre / *CDHF Tube*
25 What is a Calorie? / *Emma Bryce TED*
30 Move your Way: Play for Fun, Build Skills for LIfe / *ODPHP*
31 Kids Heart Challenge Heart Facts
/ *American Heart Association*
32 Kids Heart Challenge Main Program
/ *American Heart Association*
35 Meow Wolf Presents: Cooking with KIds New Mexico
/ *Cooking with Kids, Inc.*
36 Engaging Students to Rewrite the Recipe of School Food
/ *Healthy Schools Campaign*
37 MyPlate Kitchen link / *MyPlate.gov*
38 adapted from MyPlate.gov
39 Sugar: Hiding in Plain Sight / *Robert Lustig TED-Ed*
41 Grade 7 The Red Carpet Video / *USDA F N S*
42 What Does Sugar Actually Do To Your Body?
/ *University of California*
43 Your Food is Trying to Tell You Something / *FDA - mulitvu*
47 Cicero and the Roman Republic / NBC News Learn
49 Is it a Fruit of Vegetables? Fruits vs Veggies
/ *2 Minute Classroom*
52 How To Grow Fruit & Vegetables At Home - No Garden Necessary / *Cleverly*

53 Creating The Never-Ending Bloom / *SciF*
54 "The Magic Moment" - Peter Dahmen the Amazing Paper Engineer / *ChristopherHelkey*
58 The Beauty of Pollination - Moving Art™ / *Moving Art*
62 Potato- How Does it Grow? / *True Food TV*
69 MyPlate, MyWins: What's Your Healthy Eating Style? / *USDA*
70 How the Food You Eat Afects Your Brain
/ *Mia Nacamulli - Ted-ED*
71 The Case Crusaders Present "Portion Control & Variety
/ *HealthyUSA*
72 Welcome to MyPlate Kitchen / *Myplate.gov*
77 What a Good Night's Sleep Does for the Brain
/ *BrainFacts.org*
81 Haiku The World's Shortest Poem / *Japan Video Topics*
84 How to Slice and Mince - for Kids / *Cooking with Kids, Inc.*
86 Hack Shack- Buddy Oliver / *Jaimie Oliver*
87 Ants on a Log Snack / *SNAP4CT Recipe*
88 Discover MyPlate "Look and Cook" Recipes Video / *USDA Food and Nutrition Service*
89 Best-Ever Carrot Raisin Salad Recipe | Light & Delicious!
/ *MOMables - Laura Fuentes*
90 What's Totally Bananas and Makes for a Delicious Dessert?
/ *Kid Food Nation*
92 How to Make the Perfect Hard Boiled Egg / *Get Cracking*
93 Cooking with Kids: How to Make Deviled Eggs
/ *Fair Oaks Farms*
94 How to Make Oatmeal in the Microwave / *Quaker*
95 How to Make Easy Mexican Agua de Horchata / *Easy Green Cooking*
96 CACFP Cooking Video: Peach and Yogurt Smoothies Ages 3-5 / *USDA FNS*
97 CACFP Cooking Video: Cheesy Bean Tostada Ages 6-18
/ *USDA FNS*
98 Home Run Hummus Wraps / *Maine SNAP-ED*
99 Salsa Fresca Recipe / *Arizona Department of Health Services*
100 Stanly Tucci: How to Make Marinara Sauce / *VISCERA TV*
101 Three Sisters (Corn, Beans, and Squash) / *WisconsinDPI*
102 Simple Sautéed Spinach / *Eating Well Test Kitchens*
103 Pici Pasta | Buddy Oliver & Gennaro Contaldo / *Cooking Buddies*
109 youtu.be/eW2hYfnCfXs Homemade Chicken Nuggets | Jamie & Amber / *Jamie Oliver*
113 Eating Too Much Salt? 4 Ways to Cut Back...Gradually
/ *US-FDA*

GAME PLAN

SAFETY RULES FOR KITCHEN KIDS

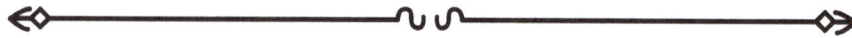

Cooking is a great life skill.
Following important safety rules prevents dangerous accidents from happening. Follow these **Basic Safety Tips** and have lots of safe cooking fun.

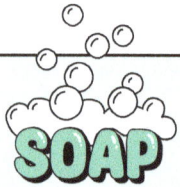

SOAP Always wash your hands with soap and warm water before starting anything. Proper hand washing keeps you from getting ill and spreading germs to others.

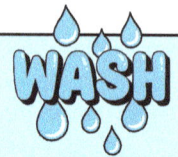

WASH All fruits and veggies. (White vinegar is great for cleaning! page 85)

RAW MEAT & EGGS
Always keep hands, dishes, tools, and cutting boards which touched raw meat or raw egg separate from all other foods. Wash everything well with soap and hot water.

TURN OFF
Always turn off the stove if you leave the kitchen. Never leave cooking food unwatched.

LABELS
Never use anything that is not clearly labeled.

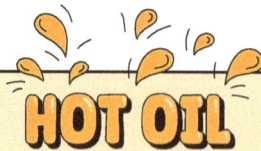

HOT OIL Never add water or liquids to hot oil. The hot oil will spit and jump at you. Someone will get burned. Always have adults do any frying in oil. Hot oil is just too dangerous to ever be worth the risk. Or maybe, skip the hot oil and try a healthier way to cook. See the cooking section for tips.

ELECTRICITY
Keep anything electric away from water. Keep wet hands away from plugs.

STAY SAFE

119

FIRE SAFETY

Keep oven mitts near the cooktop for easy access. Keep anything that can catch on fire away from the stove.

REFRIGERATE

Store cooled cooked foods in the fridge.

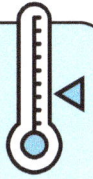

ALWAYS TURN HANDLES TO THE BACK OF THE COOK TOP

Small kids could grab the handles and others could bump into them. The hot food will fall down and someone will get burned.

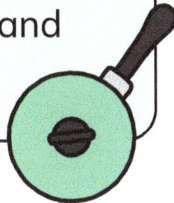

KNIVES

Never put anything sharp into a sink or bowl of water. Someone could get cut. Keep fingers away from sharp knives. Ask an adult to help you cut or slice foods that need a sharp knife.

FIRE EXTINGUISHER

Keep a working fire extinguisher in the kitchen and know how to use it.

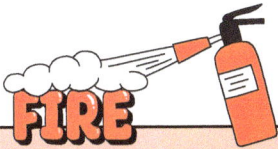

FIRE

NEVER USE WATER TO PUT OUT A COOKING FIRE.
Water makes grease fires bigger. Smother small flames with a pot lid or a layer of salt or baking soda.

IF SOMEONE GETS BURNED

Place burned area under cool running water.

DO NOT use ice or anything else.
DO NOT remove burned clothing.
DO NOT pop blisters.
GET HELP!

IN AN EMERGENCY
CALL 911
POISON CONTROL
1 800 222 1222

STAY SAFE

www.ingramcontent.com/pod-product-compliance
Lightning Source LLC
Chambersburg PA
CBHW042348030426

42335CB00031B/3499